A HYPOCHONDRIAC'S GUIDE TO

BEATING
CANCER

YOU'LL LAUGH, YOU'LL CRY,
YOU'LL CALL YOUR DOCTOR

DAVID AIZER

ISBN: 9781089157885

Imprint: Independently published

Testimonials

"Dave has been a trouper in his personal fight against melanoma as well as in his commitment to increasing awareness and fundraising in the community. He has morphed hypochondriac anxiety into purposeful action."
Jose Lutzky, M.D.
Director, Mount Sinai Melanoma Program and Chief, Division of Hematology & Oncology at the Mount Sinai Comprehensive Cancer Center, Miami Beach, Florida

"*A Hypochondriac's Guide to Beating Cancer* is a humorously insightful story of one man's roller coaster ride towards physical, and emotional, well-being. Dave Aizer captures his unique cancer journey with a storyteller's charm that is relatable for anyone touched by this disease."
T.J. Sharpe – Stage 4 Melanoma Survivor
Advocate and Author of "Patient1" melanoma blog on philly.com

"Dave is extremely committed to fighting melanoma in any way he can, and to helping others who are also fighting this deadly cancer. I am amazed by how positive and proactive Dave is despite everything he has been through. I know he will be as big an inspiration to you as he has been to me. "
Rachel Thomas – Melanoma Advocate

"Being a cancer survivor myself, I deeply appreciated David's perspective. His openness, honesty, and authenticity about the things a person thinks about before, during and after being diagnosed with cancer are so true. I LOVED his sense of humor as he described his journey. I believe that David's story and personality are exactly what's needed to give people hope and healing for themselves and their families."
Willard Barth, Author – "*The Anatomy of Transformation,*" Keynote Speaker, Executive Business Consultant & Transformation Expert

Acknowledgments

To Dr. Lee Smith, Dr. Kenneth Stein, Dr. Mark Bernhardt, Dr. Francisco Civantos, Dr. Brian Jewett, and Dr. Jose Lutzky: thank you all from the bottom of my heart for your expert medical guidance. Without all of you this book might have had a ghost writer.

To the nurses and medical staff who continue to take such great care of me. I'm not the world's easiest patient so I appreciate you very much.

To Lisa Boccard, JoAnna Tuttle, and all the other survivors I met along the way. You gave me the confidence to keep fighting each day.

To my family and friends: no man could ever have a better support system. You've been with me through the worst and the best of it. I love you all.

And last, but not least, to the mole that started it all. I can't say I miss having you around but without you I wouldn't have become the man I am. So, thank you, I guess.

Contents

"Against the assault of laughter, nothing can stand."
Mark Twain

"Laughter is the best medicine."
Unknown,
but pretty much everyone says it so it must be true

Introduction

In January of 2015 what looked to be a small, innocuous mole on my face was diagnosed as malignant melanoma and eventually became stage 3 cancer. More on that later. Through my now four-and-a-half-year journey with this disease, I have experienced every emotion in the book; specifically, in this book. So, I figured why not put it down on paper? Only problem is, what could I possibly share about cancer that hasn't already been shared? Newsflash: cancer sucks.

Then it hit me. What the world needs is a funny book about cancer because although cancer isn't particularly hilarious, some funny stuff DOES happen along the way, especially if you're a raging hypochondriac like I am. Who else would mistake a harmless eye sty for ocular melanoma or self-diagnose a foot falling asleep as a spinal tumor.

My hope in writing this book is to make you laugh, even if it's at my expense. More than that, it's to empower you to take ownership of your feelings, whether you're personally going through cancer or know someone who is. People will tell you to relax, appreciate the day, be grateful, eat kale, meditate, and a million more things, and all that may be great advice, but it doesn't change the fact that you're going through something really freaking tough. You're allowed to be scared. Besides, kale is gross.

Consider this book your permission slip to feel however you want to feel. If you want to cry: cry. If you want to be angry: be angry. By all means, if you want to laugh: laugh. I've laughed a lot in these four-and-a-half years (often at myself) and it's been really therapeutic. In fact, I credit laughter as one of the main reasons I'm now healthy and cancer-free.

And, like me, if you think every ache and pain is the end of your life, that's okay too. Whatever fear, neuroses, or hypochondriasis you're experiencing, you are not alone. It's totally normal, so don't beat yourself up over it. I have freaked out about nearly every single part of my body since my diagnosis, and I'm still here to talk about it. I'm beating cancer, and you can, too.

Just be proud of yourself for being in the fight and being a warrior. It takes guts. Oh, and by the way, I began writing this book while on vacation in Turks and Caicos. Yup, a hypochondriac who had melanoma and is terrified of the sun started writing his memoir on a beach in the Caribbean. See that, anything's possible. And if the globs of sunscreen and the layers of clothes I wore that day didn't do their job, and I end up with another melanoma that manifests in a few years, I suppose it will give me a reason to write a sequel; so, there's a silver lining. It's all about finding a positive in the negative.

Please know that nothing you are about to read has been made up or embellished. I am, in fact, this much of a basket case.

And with that: happy reading.

CHAPTER 1

One Of Many, Many Days In The Sun

It was a boiling hot afternoon in Orlando, Florida in 2001, as I hosted Nickelodeon's hit game show *Slime Time Live* on our outdoor set at Universal Studios in front of a packed audience. The show that day featured Joey Fatone and Lance Bass from *NSYNC so the energy was even more insane than usual. The crowd of kids and teens desperately wanted two things: a chance to see Joey and Lance and a chance to be slimed by me.

It seemed ironic that the *NSYNC guys dropped by that day because the temperature felt like 98 degrees (the name of a competing boy band). In addition to the sun beating down on me, studio lights and a reflector pointed directly at my face to ensure I looked my best.

I don't remember if I wore sunscreen under my makeup, but I can tell you it wouldn't have mattered anyway, because within the first 10 minutes of every *Slime Time* episode I got covered in slime and whipped cream pie. After the makeup artist would apply a wet towel to my face to clean me up, all my makeup and sunscreen would vanish.

That marked one of hundreds of episodes of *Slime Time Live* I hosted outside, in the middle of the day, in the Orlando heat, from 2000-2004. Sure it was hot, but who cared? I absolutely loved it. And I had a pretty good tan going.

Slime Time remains the longest running live game show in Nickelodeon's history, and it put me on the map; Tiger Beat, J-14, and other magazines wrote profiles about me. I partied with A-list celebrities and traveled the country, and Europe, hosting shows for Nickelodeon. I held a place in the Guinness Book of World Records for throwing the most pies and sliming the most people. I even got frosted tips on my black hair. Don't ask. It was a thing back then.

It was the best time of my life and the best gig I have ever had. My experience at Nickelodeon led to what has now become a 20-year career on television; much of it outdoors, in sunny environments, with lights and reflectors pointed at my face. In fact, I still shoot segments outside all the time—only now I apply and re-apply and re-re-apply sunscreen.

I have no idea what caused the melanoma that first appeared on my face in 2014. I don't know if it had anything to do with all the years spent outside hosting television shows or all the sports I played growing up in South Florida. There's a small chance it isn't even sun-related. It might have just been genetics. Regardless, I have definitely logged plenty of daytime hours outdoors in hot climates.

But before I tell you the story of my melanoma diagnosis, let's take a look back at my childhood and the roots of my hypochondria.

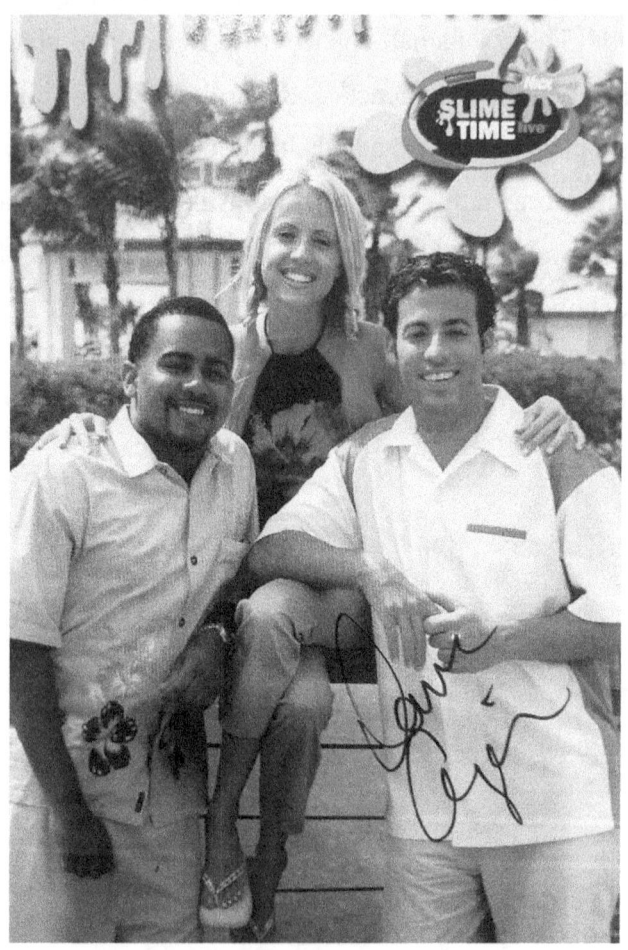

Hanging out with Jonah and Jessica, my *Slime Time* cohosts.

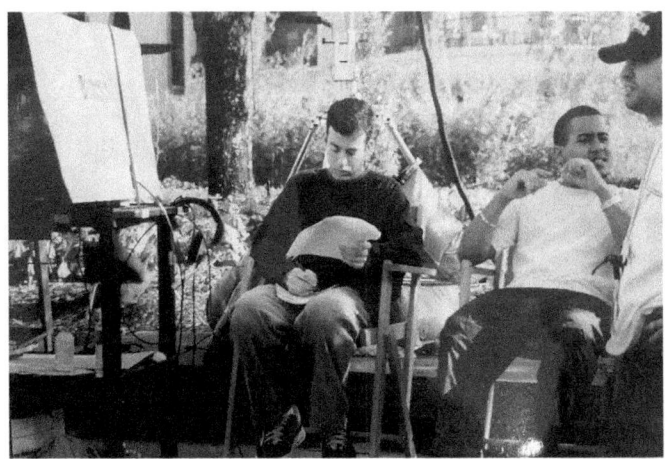

I'm rather engrossed in that script.

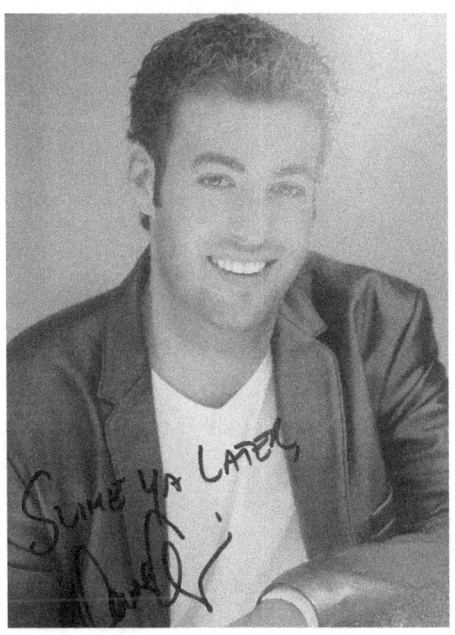

Check out the hair. Yep, that reads, "Slime Ya Later."

CHAPTER 2

Before It Began, It Had Already Begun

For as long as I can remember, even well before cancer, I have always been a hypochondriac. It might have something to do with my rather calamitous childhood. I broke my wrist and thumb playing baseball, my collarbone playing football, and my ankle playing basketball. Given all that, is it any wonder I ultimately settled on tennis as my favorite sport?

As a kid, I also broke two ribs falling out a window, broke my nose falling off a booth at McDonald's, needed the Heimlich maneuver after choking on a sandwich at summer camp, cut my eyelid on the edge of a coffee table, was bitten by my grandma's Beagle, stepped on a rusty nail (which my mom had to yank out of my foot), and more.

And to top it all off, during one particularly stressful visit to a pediatric cardiologist when I was seven, the doctor diagnosed me with a moderately leaky aortic valve, medically known as aortic insufficiency. I vividly remember that day; the cardiologist putting me through a battery of tests, then explaining to my concerned parents I might eventually need a valve replacement. That was a scary experience; my parents were worried and that, in turn, worried me.

You put all those moments together and it's easy to see how a child could become a hypochondriac. I developed a terrifying fear of doctors' offices. It's called white coat hypertension and, to this day, every time I set foot in a doctor's office my heart races and my blood pressure skyrockets.

I go to the cardiologist annually for an EKG and an echocardiogram, but my aorta has yet to present any real problems. Sometimes I get a bit short of breath and there are rare moments of lightheadedness, but generally I'm good. In fact, I've played tennis twice a week for years and done some weightlifting and my valve has held up fine. That said, the fear of my aorta exploding has tormented me, even though I'm pretty sure aortas don't explode.

And it's not just when I visit my cardiologist. It is literally any doctor's office where there's even a remote chance they might take my blood pressure—that includes the dentist, the urologist, and the podiatrist. For all I know blood pressure is highly relevant to the foot. The point is I can never relax when I go to the doctor, which is horribly inconvenient in that I've probably been to the doctor 50 times in the past four-and-a-half years. So, cancer, coupled with my fear of having my blood pressure taken, has made every doctor visit a gigantic pain in the ass.

Through the years I've also obsessed about my sexual health. Ever since I watched Magic Johnson tell the world he had HIV, I've been petrified of that disease and all the other STDs out there. There's a scene in *The Naked Gun* where Leslie Nielsen and Priscilla Presley have sex in full body condoms. If they sold those I'd probably would have bought one and suited up every time I had sex.

Back in 1992, I gave blood as a college freshman as part of the University of Miami's Greek Week activities. I'd had sex as a junior in high school and the girl bled. My first time ever and it lasted all of 30 seconds and the girl bled. Not exactly a stellar introduction into the world of lovemaking. Anyway, since that moment the idea that I'd contracted HIV from her was on my mind, and I worried I might be walking around with the disease, which at the time was a death sentence.

The weeks after I gave blood were torturous. Every walk to my dorm's mailroom caused anxiety. I prayed every day not to find a letter from the American Red Cross sitting in my mailbox. As it turned out I never got a letter from the American Red Cross; I got a personalized phone call instead. I remember sitting in my dorm room, playing Nintendo's *Tecmo Super Bowl* about a month after giving blood when the phone rang.

"Hello," I said, while trying to score a touchdown with the 49ers.

"Hello, this is the American Red Cross. Is this David Aizer?"

And with that, I dropped the Nintendo controller, Jerry Rice got tackled on the two-yard line, and my heart sank.

I told the lady on the phone it was in fact me, and she said, "Mr. Aizer, did you recently give blood?"

I heard that and thought, "This is it. I'm dying. Here's the death phone call. Why didn't I use a condom?!? I can't believe I'm going to die. I only had sex one time and it wasn't even good!"

"Yes," I replied, "I did recently give blood. Is there a problem?" By this time, I was panic-sweating.

"Well," she said, and paused either for no reason or because she's the meanest woman who ever lived, "we can't read your handwriting and aren't sure how to spell your last name."

"A! I! Z! E! R!" I replied, screaming each letter into the phone with savage ferocity. "Am I okay? Is everything okay?"

"Yes, you're fine," she said. "You're actually a universal donor, and we encourage you to donate whenever you can. Thank you."

And that was it. The American Red Cross called to tell me they couldn't spell my last name. And I haven't given them any blood since. Although now that I think about it, that's pretty selfish and I probably should.

Some years after that I kissed a girl while living in Los Angeles - just a kiss, nothing more - and woke up the next day with a cut inside my cheek and thought surely THIS was the end of me. Never mind that it was probably a canker sore or I bit my cheek during the night. No, I was convinced she had infected me with something. I didn't know what or how, but I was reasonably sure I was going to die. Perhaps she bit my cheek and her bodily fluids mingled with my blood, and now I was doomed.

Despite the fact this made zero sense, I thought about it for three months (because that's how long it took until an HIV test would be accurate) and then dragged my buddy to a mobile STD-testing van in the parking lot of a sketchy shopping center in a really horrible part of L.A. In fact, the only thing scarier than the HIV test was the van I took it in. I thought if I didn't walk in with an STD, I was leaving with one. Turns out I was fine, and my friend still makes fun of me for it.

I've also sat in movie theaters with low audio and thought I was going deaf, squinted my way through an eye exam for fear of a diagnosis of vision loss, and lost my keys and thought it was early onset Alzheimer's.

I also experienced a sleep apnea saga, which turned out to not even be sleep apnea. For two years, I woke up almost every night gasping for air, sometimes multiple times a night. At first, I assumed it had to do with my aortic insufficiency. It didn't. Then I thought my long uvula was obstructing my airway (that sounds dirty, but I assure you it's not – the uvula is the little flap of skin in the back of your mouth that hangs above your throat). That wasn't it either. I changed my diet, wore Breathe Right strips, slept on my side, slept with a wedge pillow, and meditated; nothing worked. I still woke up gasping for air.

I even took a sleep-study, which is so unbelievably weird. You're strapped to a whole bunch of wires and electrodes as three people watch you from another room while you try to sleep. I kept thinking, "They're probably running a gambling ring, taking bets as to when I'll doze off." Whoever had 4:30 a.m. was the big winner. But in the 39 minutes I slept that night I exhibited no signs of sleep apnea.

So, whatever I had it wasn't sleep apnea. It was most

probably in my head which, as you are probably gathering, is a continuing theme in my life.

Oddly enough, the thing that finally made the whole apnea situation go away was melanoma. Getting diagnosed with cancer *helped* me sleep better. I guess my brain only had room to deal with one health-related crisis, and sleep apnea got pushed to the back burner. I can't even imagine what would push melanoma to the back burner— bird flu, Zika, a flesh-eating virus?

So, you see, even before my cancer diagnosis, the pieces were in place for a major mental meltdown. And then I went to the dermatologist.

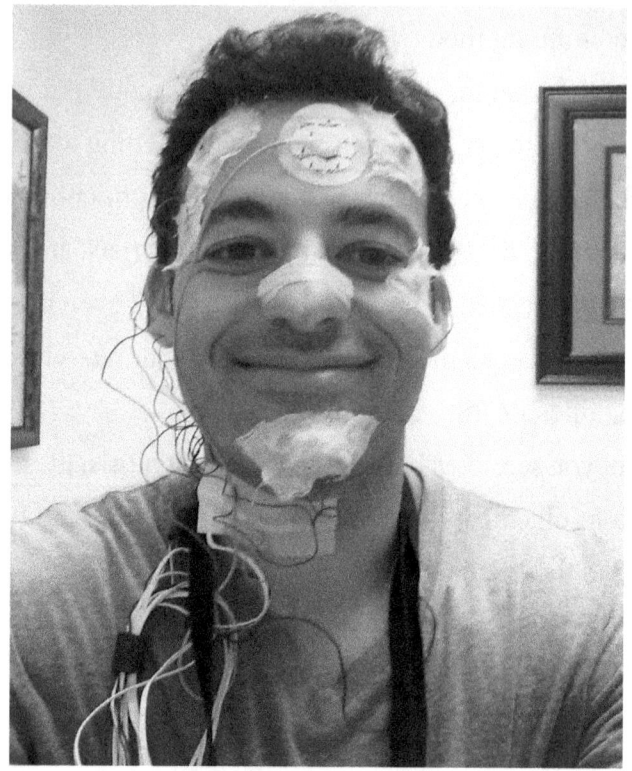

All wired up for my sleep apnea study.

CHAPTER 3

Visiting The Dermatologist

I celebrated my 40th birthday on November 24th, 2014, feeling better than ever. I was thriving in my job as a television host for WSFL-TV, the CW network affiliate in South Florida, hosting and executive producing two weekly talk shows: *Inside South Florida*, a lifestyle and entertainment show, and *Get Some*, which focused on love and dating in South Florida. In fact, I'd just received a regional EMMY nomination for *Get Some*. Plus, I'd recently hosted a series of exciting interviews, including: Phil Collins; star athletes David Ortiz, John Cena, and Steph Curry; a bevy of Miss Universe contestants; and a literal boatload of 70's TV celebs aboard a *Love Boat* themed cruise ship. I'd also participated in a professional wrestling match at a Comic Con event where I got to hit a wrestler with a chair, which was a bit of a childhood fantasy come true.

Outside of work, life was great as well. My health seemed perfect (other than the sleeping stuff), and I shared an amazing relationship with a woman I loved. We'd been dating for over a year and, although she lived in New York and we only saw each other every month or so, the times we spent together were wonderful. The plan was for her to move to Florida in the coming year. And on my 40th birthday, she and I spent the day zip lining in Belize. I felt on top of the world. Life was pretty damn good.

I'd had a mole on my left cheek for several months but hadn't really paid it any mind. But when I got back to South Florida after my vacation, I noticed in the mirror one morning that the mole looked different. It seemed to be getting bigger and when I shaved my face the mole felt bumpier than before. And then I remembered that I'd woken up two separate mornings in October with blood on my pillow; both times I dismissed it as a nosebleed or something, but now I was thinking it might have to do with my mole. So, being a hypochondriac and fearing the worst, I went to see a dermatologist. As it turned out, going to the doctor when I did paid off. It is the reason I'm alive to write this book.

This was a new dermatologist for me and I chose him simply because of his proximity to my office. Not his credentials, not his reputation, just how long it would take me to get to him. Traffic in South Florida is brutal, especially during snowbird season, and the thought of sitting in massive gridlock on my way to a doctor stressed me out almost as much as actually seeing a doctor. I mean, I love Canadians as much as the next guy, but why do they all have to vacation in Ft. Lauderdale?

Yeah, sure, there was something growing on my face, but I didn't feel like dealing with traffic to see anyone about it. Whoever the doctor was, he or she had to be close.

Thanks to Google Maps I had the good fortune of choosing Dr. Mark Bernhardt. Not only is his office only a mile from mine, but he happens to be an amazing physician, and he's been with me every step of the way. In fact, I've sent so many people to Dr. B that if he ever buys a yacht he should name it after me.

When I walked into Dr. Bernhardt's exam room he almost immediately said to me, "Tell me about that mole on your face." I knew right then and there I had a problem.

It's important to take a step back and mention that I had been to a different dermatologist's office about six months before that. I had used that dermatologist for years and felt comfortable with him, but on that day, I never got to see him. I saw his physician assistant instead. She looked at the mole, dismissed it as cosmetic, and told me I had nothing to worry about. Then she wished me well and that was the end of my visit.

Perhaps at that time the mole wasn't yet melanoma. It might have been pre-cancerous or not cancerous at all. Or, perhaps it might in fact have been melanoma, and if the dermatologist had seen me he would have been more aggressive and biopsied it and it may never have spread.

At this point, it doesn't really matter. I don't want to live in the past. But I will say, as a patient, you should ALWAYS see the physician. Even if the people at the doctor's office tell you he or she isn't available. It's your right.

I did call the original dermatologist's office after my diagnosis to let the doctor know I had melanoma. The office manager pulled up my chart and told me she saw no record of the mole from my last visit. I countered by saying that didn't surprise me, it was dismissed as "nothing." The manager then expressed her sympathies for me and told me if I ever wanted to come back as a patient they would be happy to see me.

"No thanks," I said, "I'll pass."

I wouldn't go back there if I had a mole literally on fire. Plus, that office is like an hour away.

But back to my new dermatologist, Dr. Bernhardt, one of the men to whom I owe my life. He's Ivy League educated, has an incredible bedside manner, and is a funny dude. The waiting room is unlike any I've ever seen in a doctor's office. It has a nautical theme, with multiple metallic fish sculptures hanging from the ceiling (think Jacque Cousteau's man cave). In fact, the whole place has a very retro, homey kind of vibe. For a guy who hates being in doctors' offices, this is as good as it gets. To put it simply, Dr. B is my guy. If he told me to dip my skin in a vat of wax I'd probably do it. I trust him unfailingly.

Dr. Bernhardt suggested we biopsy the mole. I fought him on it; I think in part because I had a really bad feeling and didn't want to find out the truth. But, thankfully, we proceeded. He removed the skin tissue, examined the rest of me, sent the tissue to the lab, and we parted company. And then about two weeks later, in early January 2015, he called me.

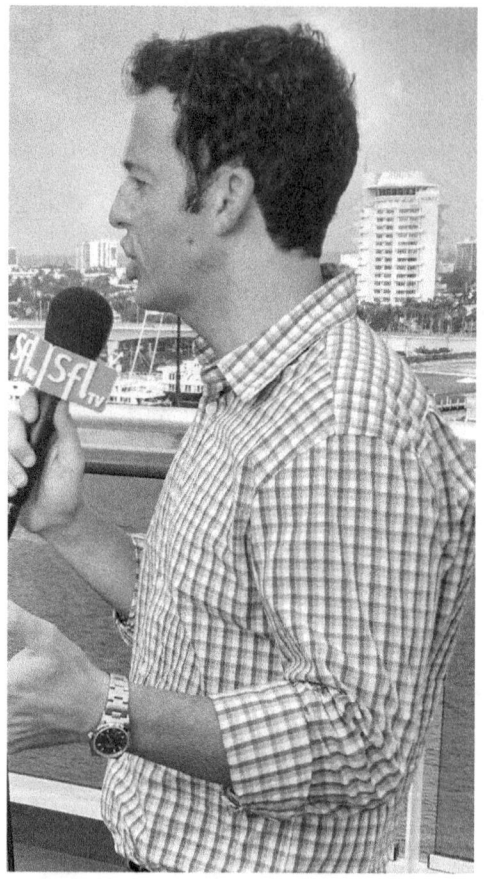

There it is. I had no idea that tiny thing could kill me.

CHAPTER 4

The Phone Call That Started It All

Through my entire melanoma saga, I've had a few phone calls that started with, "Mr. Aizer. This is Dr...." I can tell you that is usually a bad sign. When awaiting medical results, you want to hear from the nurse. Nurse = good news. Doctor = deep trouble.

When I got the call from Dr. Bernhardt on January 5th, in the parking garage at my office, I knew it wasn't to ask how my New Year's Eve went. I'd just finished rocking out to Bon Jovi as I walked from my car to the elevator, ready to conquer the workday when the phone rang.

"Mr. Aizer," he said, "it's a good thing we removed that mole when we did because it's malignant melanoma."

He went on to explain that it was small, and we caught it early, but I needed to have it surgically extracted. All I heard was, "Mr. Aizer: CANCER." Not a great way to start the year.

There is something totally surreal about getting that phone call. In an instant I went from a guy who didn't have cancer to a guy who did. Everything changed, and my life would never be the same. Bon Jovi's *Livin' on a Prayer* had just taken on a whole new meaning.

I immediately called one of my closest friends, Lee Smith, who happens to be an ear, nose, and throat surgeon. My dad and Lee's dad grew up together, so I've known Lee since he was born, two years after me. He's more like a brother than a friend and has been there for me throughout this entire ordeal. I conservatively estimate that I've asked Lee 600 medical questions since my diagnosis, and he's answered them all, no matter how nonsensical they may be.

Along my journey, I have been lucky enough to have a few small miracles. Having one friend who's a surgeon and another, Dr. Ken Stein, who's my radiologist has helped me so much. They have been, and continue to be, gigantic pillars of strength and comfort.

Although if I had to guess, both of them are probably tired of me calling and asking, "Dude, my stomach hurts, has the melanoma spread to my liver?" And I'm sure they'd be happy if I stopped texting them, "Hey man, I've got a headache. Is it brain cancer?" Perhaps that's the benefit of asking these questions via the phone: I can't see them roll their eyes while smacking their foreheads with the palms of their hands.

When I called Lee, I expected him to tell me everything was going to be all right and not to panic. After all, we caught it early, and it was skin cancer, so they would just cut it out of my face and that would be that, right? I'd have a scar, but chicks dig scars. Maybe my girlfriend would find me even sexier. And perhaps it would give me some cache on TV, like Tina Fey's scar did. That's right, melanoma would work for me. I'd be sexier AND more interesting. Maybe I'd even get a national television show out of this. In your (perfectly symmetrical non-scarred) face, Ryan Seacrest!

Not so fast. While Lee didn't give me any bad news, per se, I didn't receive the warm blanket of comfort I hoped for. He expressed that I needed to see the best head and neck cancer surgeon in town—whom Lee once studied under—immediately. I've learned that when doctors say "immediately," you might want to jump on that. So, I did. And with my buddy's help I secured an appointment the next day.

To think that on December 31st I made a resolution to be better at guitar. On January 5th I made an appointment to see a cancer surgeon. Side note: I'm still not better at guitar.

I went to the surgeon Lee recommended at the University of Miami's Sylvester Cancer Center. The waiting room teemed with patients who had come from everywhere to see him, and it took three hours before it was my turn. That's three hours of looking at sick, scared, desperate people. Now I was freaking out.

When I went into meet him (after a blood pressure reading of 170/100), the surgeon broke down the melanoma's size, mitosis rate, growth pattern, and some other stuff that, at the time, went over my head. I felt overwhelmed and dizzy, but the doctor patiently guided me through it. The mole was small (less than one millimeter) but he would need to dig deep inside my face to fully extract it. He wanted to remove some surrounding lymph nodes as well to make sure the melanoma hadn't spread internally.

Although the doctor didn't like giving percentages, he estimated that, based on the mole's size, there was probably a 90% chance there was no metastasis, and I would be fine. He wanted to be aggressive and remove a few nodes, just to be certain. Despite what seemed like good news, and great odds, I started to cry. Right there in the office. I couldn't believe that I was having a conversation about cancer… and melanoma at that. I thought melanoma afflicted old people who had spent years sunbathing in tanning oil. I rarely went to the beach, and I'd never seen the inside of a tanning bed. Sure, I didn't always wear sunscreen, but I wore it sometimes. That had to count for something. How could this be happening to me?

He tried to reassure me that I would be all right. I gathered myself, forced a smile, and we set a surgery date for three weeks later. I spent those three weeks getting mentally and physically ready, and reading far too much WebMD, which is a really, really bad idea for a hypochondriac. Not only did I have melanoma, but I became convinced I had some other stuff too, like gout.

I didn't have gout, but it didn't seem pleasant.

Then it was time for surgery.

CHAPTER 5

Surgery, Part 1

The day of my surgery I felt strong—frightened something would go horribly wrong in the operating room, or my aortic insufficiency would flare up, or I'd have an adverse reaction to the anesthesia, or a nurse would drop something inside me—but strong nonetheless. Irrational fears be damned, it was go time.

The plan was for my mom to take me to the hospital and for my father and sister to arrive before I went under the knife. My brother lived in New York, but he'd be getting plenty of updates over the phone. My mom would also provide updates to my close circle of friends, via text. I have such awesome family and friends: I can't even imagine what this whole experience would have been like without them.

My mom, Iris, is pure love. She's the family's biggest cheerleader and the one you go to for a pep talk or a pick-me-up. She's the kind of woman who makes you feel better, simply by being in her presence. She's always proud of me, and my brother and sister, and sides with us unequivocally, even when we're wrong. And while she's admittedly squeamish, she's been a trooper through all this, seeing more of my blood and battle wounds than any mother should ever have to see.

But make no mistake, my mom can be tough when she needs to be. At 12-years-old, I stepped on a nail and although she didn't want to yank it out of my foot—and I didn't want her to—she looked me in the eyes and pulled that sucker out as hard as she could. In retrospect, medically that might not have been the proper protocol, but it's the thought that counts.

Whereas my mom would hug me for programming her DVR, I might actually have to *cure* cancer to earn a hug from my dad. That's not to say my father, Ron, doesn't love me—he does— it's just that he didn't grow up in an affectionate household, so he isn't the most affectionate guy. It's been a lifetime of handshakes and back pats between us, with a few awkward hugs thrown in. When the hugs do come, I try to make them count. Still though, he is my hero and always will be and I have spent my life trying to make him proud of me.

My dad is generous, humble, has a ton of integrity, and is also brutally honest. One time while watching me on live television he called during a commercial break to tell me my shirt made me look frumpy. He was right. He's also called to tell me to sit straighter and fix my hair. But I appreciate the calls—they are his way of showing love. Plus, we're concert buddies who share an affinity for rock n' roll. My dad and I have seen Axl Rose, AC/DC, Cheap Trick, Heart, Def Leppard and more. How badass is that?

My sister, Randi, is two years younger than me. While we fought incessantly as kids we're now incredibly close. Like my mom, she is pure love and very protective of all of us, but she may actually be the one person in the family, and on earth, more neurotic than me. Randi recently had a minor surgical procedure and while recuperating at home felt pressure on her bladder. Although her doctors assured her this was caused by the anesthesia, she was convinced it was going to "be like that forever." It wasn't. It was fine in two hours. Randi also used to sneak into my brother's room several times a night when he was a baby, just to make sure he was still breathing, and, in my brother's middle school years she would drive behind him while he and his friends rode bikes, even though he begged her not to do so. She's standing behind me as I write this paragraph.

Randi and her husband Reed have two adorable children, my seven-year-old nephew Easton and my five-year-old niece Minka, and they are two of my favorite people in the world. One of the reasons I was most afraid of dying was because I couldn't imagine never seeing them again, or hugging them again, or giving them piggyback rides around my sister's house. I treasure every single second I get with those kids.

My brother, Adam, is 10 years younger than me but has been my best friend since the day he was born. I used to pick him up and carry him around the house as if he were my son and although he's grown up he'll always be a "kid" to me. He and I play the same sports, root for the same teams, went to the same college, and have careers in broadcast journalism. He's one of the most successful fantasy football podcast hosts in the country. It's been tough not having Adam in Florida throughout this process, but we're all proud of the life he's built in New York. In fact, Adam and his wife Ali have a precious one-year-old son, Andrew. He's already wearing sunscreen.

So, back to the morning of my surgery. On the drive to the hospital my mom and I listened to The Howard Stern Show, which is a weirdly inappropriate thing to listen to with your mother, but it made me laugh so it served its purpose. The topic of the day was lesbian threesomes. Sorry, mom. Plus, Howard's a neurotic hypochondriac like me, so I felt like we were kindred spirits that morning. Mom and I enjoyed a soothing, stress-free, moderately awkward drive until it came time to park. I remember my mother trying to fit into a tight spot and struggling with it, over and over. She…just…couldn't…park the damn car! It felt like the universe was playing a joke on me, like, "How much more anxiety can we give this guy?" The stupid car wouldn't fit in the stupid spot. She's a good driver but, man, I was getting agitated. Normally that wouldn't bother me, but at that moment I was NOT in a good mood.

I considered grabbing the wheel and doing it myself. I mean, if we got into an accident we were at a hospital so at least we'd see a doctor quickly. But I took a few calming breaths and realized how hard this must have been for my mom. She was driving her son to his cancer operation. I'm not a parent, so I can only guess what that's like. She finally parked, and we went inside.

In the pre-op room I met with my surgeon, my nurses, and my plastic surgeon to go over the game plan. After my surgeon did his part, the plastic surgeon would take over and put me back together. Not only was I about to have major surgery, but it would be on my face, and since I made my living as a television host I worried about my career; you know, if I didn't die on the table first.

A couple of medical residents stopped in as well, to talk me through a few things and to hand me some paperwork that required my signature. One of them freaked out a bit upon realizing he used to watch me on *Slime Time Live*. Although the show ended over a decade ago, I still get recognized from time to time. Typically, not in hospitals, right before surgery, but I felt grateful for the distraction.

He asked me what slime is made of; it's a question I often get. Usually I don't tell people. I just let them guess as I smile. But screw it, for all I knew this resident might play a crucial role in my surgery. I couldn't have him mad at me, and then not hand the surgeon a critical instrument just to spite me, and then I'd die in the operating room mid-surgery…so I parted with the ingredients. Yes, my mind played out that exact scenario. And yes, it is thoroughly ridiculous, but if giving him the secret to slime somehow made my surgery a little smoother, then I'm glad I did it. Even though I'm sure it had zero bearing. Anyway, he thanked me and, while I customarily sign autographs for fans, this guy got a signed medical waiver.

After all the meetings, I took some time to collect myself. I felt ready, and excited to get this over with and get back to normal. And then just a few minutes before my surgery would begin, the surgeon came back into the room and hit me with one final bit of news that sent everything rocketing to hell.

He needed me to sign a consent form which basically indicated that if he found a huge mass while he was operating he had my permission to take it out and do whatever else was medically necessary. Wait, what? Huge mass...medically necessary...what's going on here? I thought this was going to be your run-of-the-mill "minor" cancer surgery.

The conversations earlier that morning centered around removing the rest of the mole, getting clean margins, taking out a handful of lymph nodes, and doing a bit of plastic surgery; then waking up, recuperating overnight, and going home. Now, right as I'm about to go under the knife, we're talking about a potential massive tumor and the possibility of major life-saving surgery? As the kids say, "Shit just got real."

Side note: do the kids still say that? Sometimes I need a translator to understand my millennial coworkers. Apparently, I'm not hip. Although they don't say "hip" anymore, either. But I digress.

I started crying again, weeping openly in the pre-op room in front of my mom and my doctors and nurses. All while wearing a hospital gown. Not exactly my match. com profile picture. Incidentally, speaking of dating, my girlfriend didn't fly down for the surgery; she couldn't get away from her job, which led to a huge fight that was a nice little source of bonus aggravation added to my heaping stew of angst.

For the first time I truly felt like I might die. Not the hypochondriac's version of dying when you always think you're going to die. This time it was legit. Like there *might actually be* a big mass of cancer in my body. Even in my darkest, most neurotic moments over the past few weeks when I'd let my mind go to some bad places, I don't think I ever truly believed I had a big mass of cancer floating around my body. Now, hearing a doctor say it was a possibility made it incredibly real.

And in that moment my thoughts legitimately turned to dying on the table. If I did indeed have a mass I assumed the surgery would become more complex, and with that, more dangerous. What if something went wrong and then, as we've all seen on television, things spiraled downward? As ridiculous as it sounds, I began thinking about *ER* and *Grey's Anatomy* and all those medical shows where surgeries started out normal but then there were complications, all hell broke loose, and the patient died on the table. "How to Save a Life" by The Fray (the ultimate *Grey's Anatomy* ballad) played in my head.

It's surreal to think you might go to sleep and never wake up. I know some people say they would rather die that way, but not me. I would rather see it coming, because maybe there would be something I could do about it. It's that feeling of relinquishing total control that terrified me, and probably the reason many people are afraid to fly. My doctors were about to put me under, and there wasn't a damn thing I could do about it, and the chance existed I might never wake up. I might never say goodbye to my friends and family; other than my mom. I began to process that these could be the last few minutes of my life, and they'd be spent in a hospital room, of all places. And physically I felt fine; which made the whole thing seem really unnecessary and even harder to swallow.

Now years later, with all I've been through, I have more peace when it comes to relinquishing control and allowing my faith to take over and guide me. That was a big part of my emotional healing. More on that later. But back then, in the beginning of my cancer journey, I couldn't handle "letting go" at all.

I also thought about this: if I did survive but the doctors found a mass, what would I being waking up to? My parents standing over me, devastated? Perhaps it would be my doctor, delivering the grim prognosis, while nurses stood by to comfort me? I wasn't sure if I was more worried about dying during surgery or waking up to bad news. I was scared and really sad. "How to Save a Life" reached a crescendo inside my head.

So, like any rational human being I planned my escape. I wanted to leave that hospital: STAT. But how would I do that? Create a diversion? Pull the fire alarm? I needed to find a way out of there. This was full-fledged desperation mode, something had to be done. But as I scanned the escape routes Jason Bourne style, I saw an elderly woman smiling as she got ready for her surgery. Maybe her smile was due to a profound inner-peace or maybe it was from all the drugs. Maybe she was so loopy she thought she was at the fair. Who knows? It simultaneously inspired and emasculated me…mostly emasculated. Regardless, it worked. I manned-up, dried the tears from my face, composed myself, said goodbye to my mom, had a quick chat with the big man upstairs, got an injection, and went to sleep.

I woke up about eight hours later, thrilled to be alive. I did a quick check of my body, everything seemed to still be there. I looked around, soaking up as much ambience as I could to ensure I wasn't dreaming. My plastic surgeon stood over me, the bearer of *good news.* From his perspective, everything went well with no complications.

I was groggy but thrilled to hear it. A resident dropped in to tell me the doctors didn't see any additional cancer when they opened me up, but before I could rejoice he made sure to remind me that it didn't mean there wasn't some microscopic disease in the eight lymph nodes they removed. We'd have to wait on the pathology to know for sure. Way to ruin my buzz, dude. Where's the guy who used to watch me on Nickelodeon? Is he off making slime? I liked him better.

My heart valve held up fine, I didn't experience any apnea-related drama, and the nurses all said mine was the biggest penis they'd ever seen. Okay, I made that last part up. My mom popped in to say "hi" and told me the rest of my family was outside. The girlfriend sent me some sweet texts. I survived a cancer operation. I felt good.

The rest of the night, as I lay in the hospital bed, my biggest concern centered around peeing in that stupid jar, the one with the measurements on it so the nurses can monitor your urine output. Apparently, you can't leave if you don't pee, and if you don't pee they stick the catheter back inside you. And that did not sound good. Around 4:00 a.m., with still no signs of urine, it was getting to be mission critical. I had a strong hunch I wouldn't enjoy the nurse sticking the catheter back in me, so that was not an option. I needed to pee, even if it meant bursting a blood vessel from straining.

So, I hunched over, on my knees, in my hospital bed, with the curtain drawn, trying desperately to urinate. I thought of rushing water and rainstorms, but nothing worked. I tried to tickle myself, which is one of the weirder things I have ever done. I blame that on the medication.

I even tried talking to my penis. "Damn you, make it rain. Give daddy a sprinkle." But it didn't oblige. There was a drought down below, with all signs pointing toward painful catheter insertion. Which, by the way, sounds like a topic on The Howard Stern Show.

And then, an hour or so later, when all hope seemed lost, and I resigned myself to the impending catheter, sweet heavenly relief. This time, with the curtain wide open, in full view of the other recovery room patients and all the medical staff, the heavens opened, and I let loose with a barrage of urine. Not quite a barrage, more like a smattering, but enough to get the job done. And if anyone got a peepshow, good for them; at that moment I could not have cared less.

I went to sleep, woke up a few hours later, got instructions on how to treat my wound and empty out the drain that would be stuck in my head for the next few days, and left the hospital. I was banged up, but not broken. I'd have the clean pathology report in a week or two and that would be that. A tough chapter in my life, but all things considered it could have been worse.

Little did I know it would get worse.

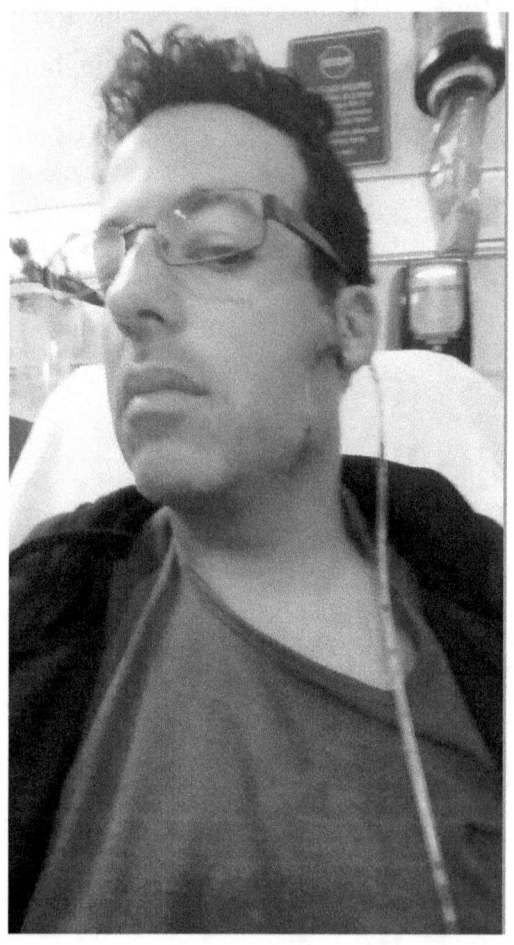

Post-surgery: bruised and battered, but feeling okay.

CHAPTER 6

From Super Bowl To Stupor Bowl

February 1, 2015 was Super Bowl Sunday. Nearly two weeks after my surgery, I still hadn't received the pathology report. I called the surgeon's office twice in that time, but no reply. Any cancer patient will tell you that waiting for medical results is the worst part because you feel helpless and your mind goes to a million different places.

Why is this taking so long? Clearly the results are bad, and they're checking it again to be sure. Is it worse than they thought? Is it some super strain of cancer they've never seen before? Are they waiting until a rabbi has office hours, so he can call me personally? I'm a good guy. I pay my taxes. Why won't anyone talk to me?

Then around 11:00 a.m. that morning, my surgeon called from his cell phone with an update. I want to mention here that I absolutely think the world of this man. Had he not chosen to be so aggressive with my surgery and remove the lymph nodes surrounding the melanoma, there's a decent chance I wouldn't be on this planet right now. Not only that, but he often called me on his own personal time, and never rushed me off the phone, and I'm not sure how many physicians would do that.

He, along with my dermatologist, plastic surgeon, and oncologist (whom you'll meet later), are the men who saved my life and continue to make sure I remain alive. I am forever indebted to each of them and would recommend them all without hesitation.

However, this, as it turned out, would be the first of two unfortunate phone conversations my surgeon and I would have.

The call consisted of good news, that was also confusing news, that would turn out to be bad news the following day. Got all that? My surgeon called to tell me that while he still didn't have the final pathology, he had the preliminary report, and everything looked clean. No indication of cancer in the eight lymph nodes the medical team extracted!

The way melanoma typically works is that it first goes to the surrounding lymph nodes and from there it spreads like wildfire to fun places like your brain, lungs, liver, and bones: you know, nowhere important, nothing you really need. But in this case, all the lymph nodes seemed to be clean, which meant an overwhelmingly great chance there was no spread. This was, obviously, amazing to hear, and a huge relief. I literally felt the tension escape my body and for the first time in over a month I could breathe without what felt like an elephant sitting on my chest.

That feeling, however, turned out to be short-lived. In fact, it lasted for a grand total of one sentence, until his next sentence began, and I'm paraphrasing here, with something to the effect of, "One part of the report is listed as incomplete, but it may just be the way it's formatted and I'll have the final results for you tomorrow."

This part is hard to explain, in fact I still don't fully understand it, but essentially one group of lymph nodes didn't have final clearance. My surgeon didn't think I should be concerned; he was optimistic those lymph nodes were negative as well, although he couldn't say with 100% certainty. In fact, after much pressing from me because I HAD to know percentages, he reluctantly offered that based on the report he was 99% confident I would be fine. He wished me well, told me to enjoy the day and the Super Bowl, and he would call me tomorrow with the final pathology report. As we hung up, I had what felt like a million different emotions running through my head. Relief, elation, gratitude, and overwhelming joy were the immediate ones, but they soon gave way to confusion, trepidation, and pessimism.

Why wasn't the report finalized? Were they running more tests? Did they take lunch and forget to finish everything? Why couldn't I just have closure.

Still, according to my doctor, my odds improved from 90% before the surgery to 99% at that moment and that would have to do until tomorrow. I sprinted out of my bedroom in my parents' house (where I spent the weekend) to tell my entire family I was cancer-free. I called my girlfriend, texted my buddies, and even sent out some emails; I did everything short of hiring a skywriter.

And I *did* enjoy the Super Bowl; except the Patriots beat the Seahawks on a last minute, game saving interception. And since I grew up a Jets fan and had recently starting rooting for the Dolphins, I hated the Patriots twice as much as I used to. It figured they would crap all over my good day.

Though as it turned out that good day ended up being not such a good day after all.

The next morning, I went to the television station, to produce a movie review segment for the upcoming episode of *Inside South Florida*. My face was still rather swollen, so I couldn't be on camera yet, but I felt pretty confident that once the swelling subsided I could hide most of my scar with makeup and my career wouldn't suffer. I really looked forward to resuming that part of my life and now that this cancer stuff seemed to be finished I could shift my focus to healing and hosting. I just needed the all-clear from my surgeon.

When my phone rang, I recognized my surgeon's number and I knew this was it: the phone call with the final pathology report. This would take me from 99% cancer-free to 100% cancer-free. Here we go!

"Mr. Aizer," my surgeon said, except he pronounced it 'Izer,' so things didn't start well.

"Hi, doc," I replied.

"Are you driving?" he asked.

"No," I replied, a little nervously. *Why would he ask me that?*

"Are you sitting down?" he asked.

"No," I replied again, and I knew I was in trouble. Nobody ever needs to sit down for good news. It's not like, "Please sit down, you've won Powerball."

The doctor told me he did have the final pathology report and, unfortunately, it wasn't good. As it turned out the preliminary report was incomplete because the lab had to run more tests, and those tests came back positive. I had cancer and it was spreading.

Just like that; the worst news I ever heard. Yesterday I didn't have cancer. Today I did, with 100% certainty. I felt as if the doctor reached through the phone and ripped my guts from my body. The cancer had spread to three of my lymph nodes and, perhaps, elsewhere. I definitely had *it*: the dreaded "C" word, in three lymph nodes. And we had to do something about *it* as soon as possible.

The doctor told me I needed another surgery on my face and neck and this operation would be massive, and the stakes would be much higher.

He apologized for calling me the day before, we spoke briefly about five-year and 10-year survival rates (always a fun conversation), set an appointment to meet at his office the next day, and said our goodbyes.

I set the phone down, closed the door to my office, and cried...again. In 24 hours, I had gone from hearing I was cancer-free to hearing my cancer had spread. That's a range of emotions I wouldn't wish on anybody.

Not only that, but now I would have to tell my family, girlfriend, friends, and colleagues the bad news; all the people I had just told I was going to be fine. It's a good thing I didn't hire that skywriter. That would have been embarrassing.

I left work, called the girlfriend, and drove to my parents' house to tell my family. What an awful day—a bunch of us sitting around trying not to think that I might die. Everybody wanted to say the "right thing" but, honestly, what can you say? We were all stunned.

But we resolved to fight the cancer as best we could, and later that night I discovered the sweet, soothing relief of a little helper named Xanax. Xanax and I would develop a nice, doctor-approved, non-addictive relationship over the next couple of years.

CHAPTER 7

A Stage 3 Diagnosis And Some Awkward Interactions

My parents and I went to see my surgeon the next day. He guided me through what the next few weeks would be like. I'd need a full body PET (positron emission tomography) scan to make sure the cancer hadn't spread anywhere else. I'd need to meet with oncologists to figure out a treatment plan after my surgery. And, speaking of that surgery, here's what it would entail: a neck dissection (meaning I would lose almost all the lymph nodes in the left side of my neck) and a parotidectomy (meaning I would lose the parotid gland from the left side of my face).

And the chance existed my facial nerve would get severed during the surgery, which could mean facial paralysis. *And* even if that didn't happen I would still need plastic surgery while I was under the knife if I ever wanted to be on TV again. *And*, for one final bit of good news, he shared with me my staging.

I had stage 3 cancer.

Officially, the diagnosis was stage 3a because the cancer found in my lymph nodes was microscopic. Stage 3a is better than 3b or 3c; but it was still stage 3 and last time I checked there were only four stages.

For some reason I had assumed it would be stage 1 cancer. Hearing the words "stage 3" felt like hearing the words "buried or cremated?" Mr. Xanax and I would hang out again right after my appointment.

Now, while this news devastated me, technically—at that moment—I might already have been completely cancer-free. Confusing, I know, but follow along: the three nodes that tested positive for cancer were the closest nodes to the melanoma and since they were now gone all the cancer *might* be gone with them. So, the option of not having a second surgery existed.

Of course, in that scenario, if other nodes in my neck did in fact have cancer and we didn't remove them I could wake up one day with a giant tumor. And by then it would probably be too late to save me. And I couldn't rely on the upcoming PET scan to tell me with certainty I didn't have cancer, since any remaining disease might have been too small at that moment to be seen.

So, I could play Russian roulette, hope the cancer was already gone, and not have the surgery *or* have a massive surgery to remove all the nearby melanoma landing spots and increase the chances of the disease being gone; but risk facial paralysis. I longed for an option "c" because both of those options really sucked.

Being a hypochondriac, I knew if I didn't have the surgery I'd wake up multiple times a night, probably every night for the next five years, to touch my neck. And I'd run to the mirror first thing every morning looking for lumps. God forbid I ever got a sore throat and swollen glands. I'd probably operate on myself with scissors and peroxide. So, I decided on surgery.

We set a date and I embarked upon a series of oncology meetings which included various estimates as to the likelihood the cancer had spread and if I would even be alive in five or ten years to talk about it. Plus, I began looking into new careers in case I emerged from my surgery deformed. Chicks may dig scars, but TV viewers, and TV executives, aren't fans of caved-in faces and necks.

Broadcasting was the only career I had ever known. I'm not particularly handy, my español es muy malo, and becoming a tennis instructor meant far too much time in the sun. I explored some radio jobs, but I began to think facial deformity might lead to me working in a carnival, or maybe I could star in a community theater production of *Phantom of the Opera*. I figured I could always get a job at a haunted house scaring kids on Halloween.

And this all went down while I dealt with the residual physical pain from my first surgery.

It was officially, or unofficially (I don't think there's a governing body for these things) time to start telling people about my cancer. I had a legit scar on the side of my face and some major post-op swelling, and I was determined to start going out again because frankly I needed laughter and alcohol, so people were going to take notice. There was no way around that.

My first night out, I went to a bar in Ft. Lauderdale called The Royal Pig. This turned out to be a Royal Pain in the Ass. It was hot and crowded, and I kept covering my face for fear of an errant elbow. Not to mention I had begun the exhausting process of checking my neck and armpit glands for swelling every five minutes, so I could self-diagnose if my cancer spread. A process which, over four years later, I'm proud to say I only do once or twice a day. Granted, I only have glands in one side of my neck thanks to my second surgery, so there isn't as much to check.

I sat at the bar, shielding my face from elbows with

one hand and examining my neck and armpits for swollen glands with the other. It's a good thing I wasn't trying to meet a woman. Unless a lady had a visual impairment or dug charity cases I don't think I was scoring any digits.

And then a woman I had known since college approached.

"Dave," she said, "how are you? What happened to your face?"

"Hi," I replied, "I'm alright, but I had surgery to remove a melanoma from my face and neck. I actually need another surgery."

I expected her to say something to the effect of, "That's horrible. Are you going to be okay? How do you feel?" Or perhaps she'd be more comforting and simply say, "It doesn't look that bad. The surgeons did a great job, and I'm sure the next surgery will be the same."

Instead, she immediately turned pale and uttered the following: "Oh, my God, Dave, my husband died of melanoma. It started out as a lump in his chest and it went to his brain. I'm so sorry."

Yup, there it was, the first of what would turn out to be multiple conversations over the next few years that essentially went: "Oh my God, my friend/cousin/father/mother/teacher died of melanoma. It started at x and it spread to their y and z. It's such an aggressive cancer. I'm so sorry, Dave."

To be fair, she felt worse about saying it than I felt about hearing it. Or maybe we tied; we both felt awful. I do think that whenever people tell me some version of that, they're trying to be helpful and sympathize, if not empathize, with me. But a note to all of you who may want to express the same sentiment to a cancer patient: please don't. It's hard for us to hear that someone you know died of our disease.

Any optimism I had been able to muster vanished at The Royal Pig that Friday night. I now knew someone who knew someone who died from my disease. And that someone who died was younger than me when it happened.

So much for the whole, "Sure people die from this but those are older people without good immune systems." Nope, this wasn't some 85-year-old, this guy was a young man, younger than me, when he passed.

Here's a sampling of some other awkward conversations I've experienced:

A friend of mine who cuts hair said her mom died from melanoma. As she cut her mom's hair, she saw a mole on her scalp, and implored her mom to go to the doctor. By then it had spread to her brain and her lungs and she soon died. I didn't even get a free haircut out of that exchange.

A waitress who dropped off guacamole at my table also dropped this bit of distressing news into my lap after hearing me say the "m" word: her dad used to own a boat, he tanned a lot, one day he had a mole, it soon spread to his liver, then he died. So much for my ahi taco.

My father's friend told me about a buddy of his who often drove with his left arm exposed to the sun, resting against the lowered window. He got melanoma on his arm, it spread to the lymph nodes under his armpit and into his brain, and he died a horrible death.

Everywhere I turned people scared the crap out of me. But despite all these interactions, or perhaps for some weird reason because of them, I found myself bringing up my cancer in conversations if people didn't bring it up first. I HAD to talk about it; all the time, to everyone. It consumed me. It felt disappointed if people didn't want to talk about my face. I'd even lean towards them, favoring my left side, so they'd hopefully catch a glimpse.

Why I did this I'm not sure. I think I just desperately needed to hear a positive story about someone surviving melanoma—just one bit of positivity that I could hold on to and keep with me. Or maybe I genuinely wanted to educate people about skin cancer, even if they didn't want to be educated.

Shortly after my diagnosis my buddy Dean took me shark fishing to try and get my mind off things: not a great fit because I get violently seasick, but I was in serious bucket list mode. I spent the day alternating between dry heaving, applying sunscreen, and lecturing everyone on the boat about the dangers of sun abuse. That included the captain, his first mate, and Dean's buddy. I can only imagine what they all thought of me. Side note: we did catch a nine-foot bull shark. Or at least that's what they told me while I leaned over the side of the boat vomiting.

My need to educate knew no boundaries. Once I walked past a tanning salon, but couldn't help myself, so I walked back over to it and went inside. A young girl, probably no more than 18 or 19, worked the front desk alone.

"Hi," she said, oozing sweetness and innocence. "Do you want to use one of our tanning beds? We have some great options."

"No thanks," I replied, and continued condescendingly. "Let me ask you something. If people ask you if these tanning beds are dangerous what do you tell them?"

This poor girl did not expect that and had no idea how to respond. After looking around desperately for help, but finding none, the best she could offer was, "We just tell them that the beds are no more dangerous than the sun."

"That's not true," I laid into her, "they're way more dangerous. You need to get your facts straight and do your research if you're going to work here."

"I'm sorry," she said, and I thought she might cry.

"Whatever," I replied, and left like a self-righteous cancer-crusader.

Not my finest moment. In fact, a low point. But I felt angry and scared and didn't want anyone else to go through this. Tanning beds are extremely dangerous and can significantly increase your likelihood of getting melanoma. Look it up and see for yourself. And I hated that I kept seeing them in strip malls, with beautiful women and men with perfect tans on posters and placards outside the storefronts.

I also felt bitter because I had never once been in a tanning bed, and yet I ended up with cancer while all these South Florida sun worshippers and tanning bed enthusiasts walked around cancer-free. It wasn't fair.

On another occasion I rolled my window down at a red light and called a homeless man over; not to give him money but to make sure he had on sunscreen. Take a guess where sunscreen fell on his priority list. I think his exact words were, "I just want a burger."

And there was the time I went to the grocery store to buy sunscreen. I should own stock in multiple sunscreen companies I've bought so much. After I picked my SPF-30 off the shelf I noticed the lady next to me had grabbed an SPF-8. I tried to mind my own business, I really did, but she needed to know that wouldn't cut it.

"Excuse me," I said, "I'm a bit of an expert on sunscreen." I'm not actually an expert, but I know SPF-8 is far too weak.

"Really?" she said, confused as to why some random guy decided to chat with her.

"Yes," I added, "I had melanoma."

That, by the way, is such a weird thing to say to someone, unsolicited, at the grocery store. Try telling a stranger buying cigarettes that you had lung cancer. See where that gets you.

Anyway, I kept the train rolling. "You need at least an SPF-30 and it has to be broad spectrum, UVA and UVB."

For once, somebody seemed genuinely happy to hear my opinion. She asked which brand I was buying, I pointed to the one on the top shelf, and she reached for it, thanked me and wished me well. I walked away feeling proud that I may have saved somebody's life. Unless of course she put the SPF-30 back, grabbed the SPF-8 and tanning oil and made a break for it.

But no conversation I have ever had has been as awkward

as the one I had with a customer service representative from JetBlue. The lack of having my girlfriend in town really wore on me. She was in New York, but she might has well have been on another planet. She seemed a million miles away. Going to bed alone every night, waking up alone every morning, seeking comfort through a telephone; it all really depressed me.

I decided to fly her in for a long weekend, but the prices were exorbitant. JetBlue is my favorite airline, and their customer service is top notch, so I figured I'd give them a call to see if I could get a better price.

After it became clear that the prices over the phone exceeded those on the internet, I tried, for the first time ever to play THE CANCER CARD. Because if you can't play the card from time to time what's the point of having cancer? I explained to the gentleman that I needed my girlfriend to come to town because of my upcoming cancer surgery, and I couldn't go through this without her. I begged him to find a way to reduce the fare; you know, as a courtesy to a cancer patient. He seemed genuinely concerned and promised me he would go check. He asked if I'd wait on hold.

When he came back, about a minute later, he said this: "Um, sir, um, okay so I asked around…is it…um…terminal?"

What?!?! I did not expect *that*.

"I don't know. I hope not," I said.

"Oh, well, um," he added, "if it was then we could probably discount the rate, but, now, um, we won't be able to do that."

I was mortified. Later, I imagined what this poor guy must have gone through when he put me on hold, and I got quite a laugh out of it. I pictured him asking his coworkers for advice, and the conversation going something like this:

"Hey, I got this guy on the phone and he's looking for a reduced fare. Apparently, he has cancer and he wants to fly his girlfriend in before he has surgery."

"Is he going to die?"

"I don't know."

"Well ask him, because if he is going to die we can probably shave a few bucks off the price."

"Seriously, I have to ask him that?"

"Yes, you do, Roger, if he wants the discount."

I don't remember if his name was Roger, it just seems like it should be. Needless to say, I didn't get the discount. I paid in full and got no benefit from playing the cancer card. I wonder what would have happened if I *had* said I had terminal cancer. Would he have asked me to send him my CAT scans? Would he want a piece of the original mole?

My girlfriend did come, on a full-priced ticket. And we had a nice weekend, although I spent the majority of it freaking out, because on Monday I would get the results of the PET scan I had taken Thursday.

At one point during the weekend we walked along the beach (I wore long sleeves, socks up to my knees, and applied half a bottle of sunscreen) and happened upon a shirtless, bronzed beachgoer in a Speedo. He was under the influence of something way stronger than alcohol and rambling incoherently. I noticed he had an enormous mole on his arm and I mentioned it to him, because, you know, that's what I did. He told us that doctors had warned him about that mole years ago, but he stopped going to doctors, because they didn't know anything, and it's all a conspiracy, and they just want our money, and who needs them. Welcome to South Florida, ladies and gentlemen!

Fair enough. I do wonder what has become of that man, and his mole, and his Speedo. Well, maybe not his Speedo.

Then on Sunday my girlfriend got an email from the airline notifying her they canceled her flight and booked her on a flight to New York Monday afternoon. This was a blessing from God; she could now be here when I got the results of my scan Monday morning.

But she missed her dog and didn't want him spending

another night without her. He wasn't in a kennel or anything; she had dropped him off at a friend's apartment. Still, she felt she needed to leave Florida Sunday, so she could get back to him. We got her on a flight that night and she left. To her, she was a dedicated mother to her pet. To me, she chose her pet over my PET scan. It was only a matter of time before this relationship, the one I thought might lead to marriage, would end.

CHAPTER 8

Healthy Living (More Or Less) And My Angel

Monday morning arrived and at approximately 9:00 a.m. and 12 seconds I called the University of Miami's oncology office for the results of my PET scan. I could have called right at 9:00, but, come on, that would be crazy. This was a huge phone call; it's one thing to have cancer in three lymph nodes, but if it was spreading throughout my body all the neck surgery in the world wouldn't save me. I remember imagining very vividly in that moment a surgeon cutting my skull open with a drill. I got the oncologist on the phone, while wondering if brain surgery would be in my future.

There are few things scarier than waiting in silence as a doctor checks the results of your exam on their computer while you try to analyze their breath sounds and the pace at which they click their mouse. As the moments ticked by I freaked out internally.

Those were some fast clicks, probably good news. Wait, why hasn't he clicked in five seconds? Is he reading something twice? It must be my liver. He's probably working his way down my body, and I feel like we are in the mid-stomach region. Wait, why is my stomach bothering me? Yup, it's my liver. Ow my stomach! Is my liver in my stomach? ...Oh wait, he clicked again. Where are we now, the groin? I can't have penis cancer! Is that a thing? Are they going to operate on it? Will I lose it? Do I man scape first? ...Ok, we're at the legs. Fast clicks, good. Can you get cancer in the leg? What about the feet? I did notice a mole on my foot. Oh, man, I have foot cancer.

As I sat on the floor in my office having this conversation with myself, while the doctor processed my results, I prayed. You know the prayer; we've all done it: "Dear God," it starts, "please let me be okay. In return, I promise I will never (fill in your own personal blank) again." In my case I chose "lie out in the sun again."

And then, the long wait mercifully ended with wonderful news. The scan turned out negative, all clean, no sign of spread anywhere! Not the lungs, not the liver, not the bones, not the penis, not the brain.

Except, wait, he's not 100% sure about the brain. Wait, what?

Apparently, a PET scan is super accurate everywhere but isn't the best indicator for the brain. So, just 10 seconds after reassuring me I had no signs of metastasis the doctor suggested I get a brain MRI, to rule out brain cancer. I needed a brain MRI after undergoing all this PET scan drama? Come on! Give a guy a break. Why do doctors always need to qualify things? Can't I just not have cancer and never talk to any of them again? And failing that, can't I at least enjoy a victory for one lousy minute?

I ultimately decided that the brain MRI would be Tuesday's problem. On that particular Monday morning, I would indeed enjoy these results. That is one thing you learn as a cancer patient: enjoy the victories, no matter how big or small they seem. Every day you wake up is a victory. Every night you go to bed in your own room and not a hospital is a victory. Every negative scan and every positive doctor visit, all victories. And they must be enjoyed. I called my family, my friends and my girlfriend (even though I was mad at her) and shared the good news. And, the next day, scheduled the brain MRI.

The brain MRI also turned out to be negative, but in the days leading up to it, and in the days leading up to every brain exam since, I developed headaches, ringing in my ears, lightheadedness, confusion, imaginary smells, memory loss, and whatever else WebMD told me I might have if I had a brain tumor. Those are always a fun few days.

Encouraging news even appeared from unlikely sources. After an appointment with a prospective oncologist, I checked out at the front desk and the receptionist, whom I'd never met, looked up at me and said, "You're going to be okay. I know you are."

She said it with total calmness and conviction, like she absolutely knew it to be true, and it floored me. I had no idea what to say back, so I just said, "Thank you." I'm not sure if I believe in psychics but this woman seemed to know my future. I walked away incredibly comforted. I still draw from that moment when I need it.

Buoyed by all this good news and feeling better about my diagnosis I decided to start living cleaner. Now, I've never taken one illegal drug and I smoked maybe four cigarettes in high school and none since, but I do enjoy an alcoholic beverage or three from time to time. And I have often fallen under the spell of that sweet vixen Diet Coke. That evil temptress has had her hooks in me for years. So that's where I would start: giving up Diet Coke, because I sure as hell wasn't giving up alcohol. A cancer diagnosis is why God invented alcohol.

So, I kicked my addiction to aspartame and dropped

down from two diet cokes a day to two a week. I wasn't going cold turkey. I already wasn't having sex, so not getting laid AND never drinking diet soda was too much for my fragile psyche to handle. I suppose I could have been intimate with the soda can and killed two birds with one stone but that would have sent me right back to the hospital.

I heard countless pieces of advice as to how I could improve my quality of life: some solicited, some unsolicited. Yoga, meditation, acupuncture, a juice cleanse (which sounded abysmal)…it went on and on. Somebody told me to smoke weed, because it would be better for me than Xanax. Somebody else told me I'm way too paranoid to smoke weed, and it would be a disaster of epic proportions. I was inclined to agree with that person, so I passed on the grass. I could just imagine sitting on a couch, jamming out to Phish, hitting a bong and then coughing, and correlating that cough with lung cancer. What a buzzkill. Nobody wants that guy at a marijuana party. Although they probably don't call them marijuana parties; see that, I'm totally not cool enough for drugs.

So, no weed but I did hire a nutritionist, whom I subsequently fired a week later because it turns out I hate nutrition. It's not that I hate it per se, it's just that it requires SO MUCH WORK. Specifically, a lot of cooking. And that,

I hate. I figured I'd take my chances eating at restaurants. Besides, I already sort of gave up soda, isn't that enough suffering?

I remember my trip through the grocery store with the nutritionist. Bless her heart; she just wanted me to make more enlightened food choices. But WOW did none of those choices seem good; sardines, quinoa, kale…what am I, a hippie?

I did take up yoga though, which really does work, and I still do it from time to time even though I don't love it. My crow pose is no better now than when I started, and I still can't do scorpion to save my life, but yoga relaxes my mind. And I played a ton of tennis. I've always been a tennis junkie and few things got me through my cancer funk more than that sport. I played a few times a week and would have played every day if I could have. I would absolutely advise physical activity as a powerful way to deal with stress. Surely, you already know this, but I can tell you firsthand it is a lifesaver. To this day, when I am worried about a relapse, a scan, or a physical exam I do a set of pushups. I've done pushups in waiting rooms, restrooms, even elevators.

Of all the opinions and advice I got at the time, one person would enter my life whose words had a more profound effect on me than anybody else I'd ever met. Her name is JoAnna Tuttle, and I met her through a cancer support organization called Imerman Angels. The Angels pair you with a survivor of the same type of cancer you have, down to the staging and everything. From the research I had done, stage 3a melanoma could go either way. I could be here in five years, or I could not. And as a guy who lived on the pessimistic side of town, I worried each day that I wouldn't be on Earth in five years.

JoAnna lives in California so we didn't meet in person; but we talked on the phone every single day, often for over an hour. She was six years cancer-free, proof you could beat stage 3 melanoma, and was the one person I could ask anything, because she had lived the exact same thing as me. The depression, the anxiety, the manifestation of imaginary symptoms, the constant worrying; JoAnna gave me a million pieces of advice on how to cope with all of it. One of the pieces of advice I still carry with me is this: JoAnna would get very nervous before scans, as she thought about all the different parts of her body suddenly bothering her. So, she would write them all down on a chart at her house and then, after her scans came back clean, she would cross each body part off the list. I do that too, thanks to her, and it is such a cool feeling.

I finally got to meet JoAnna about a year later, when she came to South Florida on business, and we had a lovely time. I don't know if I've ever felt as immediately connected to another human being as I felt with her. She spent hours upon hours of her time talking me through the scariest part of my life, and there is nothing I can ever do to properly thank her, but I hope mentioning her in this book is a start. Thank you JoAnna, I love you!

CHAPTER 9

Surgery, Part II: No Node Left Behind

The night before my second surgery I felt awful. It might have been the combination of the coal-oven pizza, ice cream cake, and soda I gorged myself on at dinner (it seemed like an appropriate time to be gluttonous), or maybe the anxiety over what would soon come. The next day's surgery would involve the removal of almost all the lymph nodes in the left side of my neck, the removal of the parotid gland from the left side of my face, and the removal of a significant amount of fat and tissue from my stomach, which would then be used to rebuild my neck and face. This would all happen during the same operation, with my surgeon removing the nodes and parotid gland and my plastic surgeon removing the belly fat and putting me back together.

And, of course, the chance existed that some of what

they took out would be cancerous. Not cancerous enough to show up on my PET scan, but cancerous nonetheless. And that would mean spread; and with spread would come a greater likelihood of death. So, I knew, even after the surgery, there would be a lot of waiting around for more results.

Oh, and even if no disease showed up in any of the lymph nodes, I still wouldn't be out of the woods. There could be undetectable cancer in my bloodstream, just swimming around, starting to do its damage. I had years of blood tests in my future.

Not to mention the lingering concern over my facial nerve and potential facial paralysis. This was a lot of stuff to worry about. Where was that Xanax?

Around 8 p.m. the night before the surgery the diarrhea started. And boy did it start. You've heard the term "shit storm?" I believe I understand its origin. But why was this happening now, the night before my surgery? I needed sleep. Instead, I wore out a path from the couch to the toilet. Which, predictably, lead to irrational thoughts.

Has the melanoma metastasized to my colon? Or maybe it's spread to my stomach? What if I have diarrhea during the surgery? Is that a thing? I'll be out cold, but will my colon know the difference? What if it happens in the O.R.? What if it happens on my doctor? How humiliating. He might kill me on purpose.

My biggest concern shifted from living or dying to crapping on my doctors and nurses. And if I did do that, what horrible nickname would they give me? I'd be the butt of their jokes for years, pun very much intended.

I finally got to sleep because, frankly, I had nothing left in my system, and I woke a few hours later reluctantly ready to go under the knife.

The morning of the operation my family and I had the same routine in place as we did for the last one. My mom would drive me to the hospital (and be subjected to more Howard Stern) while my dad, my sister, and her husband would show up later. And they'd be joined by a few of my mom's closest friends later in the day during my surgery. A party in the waiting room, in my honor. Of course, I'd miss it, but the coolest people often miss their own parties. I heard Kanye West never attends his own parties.

I got to the hospital and nurses ushered me back to the prep room almost immediately. I had sky high blood pressure but, unfortunately, not high enough to cancel the surgery. Between my anxiety and a colon that could blow at any time I was a real pressure cooker. At least I had an hour before surgery, giving me more than enough time to collect myself and mentally prepare.

Except, about a minute later, a nurse approached to tell me they changed the schedule and I was next. Suddenly, I didn't have an hour to pray, meditate, and get my act together; I had a couple of minutes. After a quick freak-out session, I asked for a moment alone. My girlfriend couldn't come down for this surgery either, and things were essentially over between us, but I had to hear her voice. We texted a bit that morning, but I needed more. I called her to tell her I loved her and to hear her say it back, but my call went to voicemail.

She claimed later that she didn't hear the phone ring and never got the message. Maybe that's true, but in that moment, I felt alone.

I left the voicemail, hung up, and asked to see my mom one more time. It's amazing, even as a 40-year-old I still needed my mom by my side. I hope that never changes. We both said, "I love you" and at 8:00 a.m. away I went, off to get this cancer out of me once and for all.

Several hours later I woke up, completely groggy, and tried to process my surroundings. I had no idea how the surgery went but, hey, I was alive so that was a plus. Or, maybe I died and went to heaven. Bring on the virgins!

The nurse seemed content with my vitals, and as I dipped in and out of consciousness I made out the time on the wall clock. It read 10:30.

Two and a half hours, what happened? Why so quick? What went wrong?

I figured out it was in fact 10:30 p.m. and my surgery was over 14 hours long. My poor family and friends; I slept through the whole thing, but not them. I hope the hospital validated their parking.

My plastic surgeon came over to tell me all had gone well from his perspective. He explained that because I'm thin he had to make a rather long incision in my stomach to extricate enough fat for my face and neck, so I should expect to have a large scar there. Great, the one time being thin screwed me. Perhaps if I hadn't gone to the bathroom so much the night before I would have been chubbier and ended up with less of a scar. But I could handle a stomach scar. It's not like I was ever going to the beach again.

Next, a member of my surgeon's team came by to tell me everything went as planned from their perspective. They took out over 60 lymph nodes from my neck and removed the parotid gland from my face; all while avoiding cutting my facial nerve. The next step would be to biopsy everything they extracted to see if the cancer had spread. Speaking of spread, I didn't know if I crapped myself during the surgery; I thought about asking but refrained.

That's a question you don't want to hear answered "yes."

My parents came in to see me too. I apologized that the surgery took so long; like it was my fault or something. We shared a nice moment together, and they wished me a good night.

All things considered, so far so good. My heart valve held up once again, I didn't die under anesthesia, and the doctors didn't see anything alarming. I had survived two cancer surgeries. I didn't give myself any credit for that at the time, but as I look back now, that's a cool thing to be able to say. If you've had a similar experience, you should be proud of yourself and wear it like a badge of honor.

That night closely resembled my first night in the hospital, except more uncomfortable and more painful. During surgery, the doctors reopened the incision on my face from the first operation, made a four-inch incision in my neck, and an eight-inch incision in my stomach. I was a mess, for sure. And once again I had a drain coming out of my head which made sleeping nearly impossible.

Another thing that kept bothering me was that stupid machine that monitors your vital signs. In addition to all the other stuff occupying my mind, I obsessed about my blood pressure readings—and telling myself not to think about it only made me think about it more. Consider that:

I was coming off a massive 14-hour surgery for stage 3 melanoma and my chief concern was the nurses judging me for having high blood pressure. That's when you know you have an irrational need to please everybody.

Every few minutes the cuff on my arm would tighten and the machine would produce some very high numbers. And then the nurses would chat about it. At least that's what I think they were chatting about. The whole thing really pissed me off. It became so frustrating I had my nurse put a sheet over the machine, so I couldn't see the numbers. That didn't work, as I mustered enough strength in my body to remove the sheet, so I could check my own blood pressure.

You read that correctly. I was hooked up to a bunch of wires and tubes, in tremendous pain, with a drain hanging out of my head, but instead of resting I was thrashing around, struggling to take a sheet off the blood pressure machine. Surely the nurses saw this; I figured it was only a matter of time before the psychiatrist walked in.

At this rate, maybe the cancer wasn't going to kill me, but a heart attack would. It got so bad I had the nurse turn the machine around. That worked, I relaxed...and almost immediately started stressing about peeing.

Excuse me, nurse, you got anything stronger than Xanax?

Like my previous surgery, I shared a room with multiple patients while plenty of nurses and doctors came in and out. It was Grand Central Station in there. And, like before, I had a lot of trouble urinating into that stupid container. But this time I didn't care about privacy or discretion, not even for one moment. With the curtain open, the penis came out, and the show was on. I gave my guy a pep talk, he obliged, and my faucet got down to business.

A few hours later, morning arrived. A doctor examined me, and—to my surprise—told me I could leave. I assumed I would be spending a couple of nights there. Perhaps it's because I was healthy, or they were short on space, or they didn't want to see me urinate again; whatever the reason, I got to go home. I went to the bathroom to change back into my clothes and that's when I saw myself.

My face and neck were a swollen, bloody mess. A giant wound ran down my left cheek and another one ran across my neckline. My left lip and left eye sagged because my facial nerve, while not severed, had been traumatized. The drain protruding out of the side of my head and the balloon connected to it brimmed with blood. I had never looked worse. Fuck you, cancer. But I was alive and leaving that hospital.

It is weird which memories are the most vivid during your journey. For me, two of them occurred while leaving that hospital. As an orderly wheeled me through the lobby, sympathetic onlookers wished me well with their eyes. But I could feel the concern expressed on one man's face, so I looked at him and said, "You should see the other guy."

He laughed and said to me, "Good for you."

Then, as I reached the exit the orderly asked how I wanted to leave the hospital. And I said, "On my own two feet." I stood up and walked out that door, without help.

And I thought to myself, "I'm going to win this fight."

CHAPTER 10

Picturing Death While Praying For Life

I wish I could say I carried that optimism with me throughout my recovery. But at that stage of my life, my optimistic moments were fleeting. Especially during the days after the surgery, because I physically couldn't do very much. I spent most of the time on my parents' couch, healing. Pain and soreness ravaged my body. The drain hanging from my head would often jostle, causing unbearable anguish. And when I wasn't hurting, I was thinking about the impending biopsy results and how crushing they could potentially be.

During that time, I thought about death a lot, even though all the news I had at my disposal was good. I couldn't help it; my mind was working against me. I may have believed I would win the fight when I left the hospital, but the more time I spent on my couch, the more I felt the opposite. And

I didn't just think about death; I thought about dying, and what dying from cancer would look like, feel like, and even smell like. Many of us have seen someone die from cancer and that image is burned into our brains. I pictured myself heading down that same road, losing so much of myself that I would become emaciated and unrecognizable.

I imagined I would be violently ill all the time. I would smell awful. I'd be soaked in sweat only to feel ice cold moments later. I would slip in and out of consciousness, not knowing where I was and forgetting people's names. I would need to be cleaned and changed, becoming a burden on my family. In the end I would pray for death. And my niece and nephew, both very young at the time, would be left with that image of me. When they grew up they would remember me like that, if at all.

I also feared I would lose my hair, which I know is not nearly as important as everything I just mentioned (and fairly shallow) but it made me mad because throughout my television career I'd always had good hair.

I constantly looked at my face in the mirror. My lip and my eye sagged and I hated what I saw. Doctors told me my face would most likely return to normal, but I looked very abnormal. Negative thoughts suffocated me.

If I did live, would I ever get my face back? Would I ever be able to look at myself again without being reminded of what I went through, and feeling profoundly sad about it? How would other people see me? Would I be self-conscious every moment of every day for the rest of my life?

One thing was for sure: if my lip and eye didn't heal this was the end of my television career. Nobody would hire me; I was convinced of that. From the moment I first anchored the morning announcements my junior year of high school I had fallen in love with television and now, if my face didn't return to form, that career would be over.

I was missing great stuff at work, including The Miami Film Festival's Red Carpet, a charity event with Miami Heat players and my weekly talk show *Inside South Florida*. And somebody else was hosting it all. In my business, if you miss a few days and the ratings improve in your absence, people start looking at making changes. That's how cutthroat it is, and that's why television hosts rarely take sick days.

I supported the girl who was filling in for me, but I also wondered if the bosses preferred her over me. I felt relieved she wasn't a guy because that would have been direct competition for me, but I remained worried that the next time I set foot in the office it would be to collect my things. I'm not saying I wanted her to fail. Let's just say

I wasn't vigorously rooting for her success.

Things got so bad, and I grew so depressed, that after a few days I called my therapist, Dr. Ron Ellis, and he talked me through it as best he could. I had been to see Dr. Ellis a couple of times since my diagnosis and, while I found him to be a great therapist, I was not a great therapy patient. Dr. Ellis was easy to talk to and made me feel better during those visits, but I didn't stick with it because therapy made me feel exposed and vulnerable. I've always had a hard time asking for help and letting my guard down and have treated those qualities as signs of weakness, almost like they made me less of a man.

But in fact, the opposite is true. As I've learned through all of this, asking somebody for help can be a real sign of strength. Now, I ask for help – and offer help – much more frequently than before, and that has made me a better man and a better friend. We're all in this together, and whether it's cancer, family stress, or just the rigors of everyday life, teamwork is such a valuable ingredient to happiness and success. Please don't be afraid to be vulnerable to others (especially your loved ones) and don't be afraid of therapy. Not seeing my therapist more throughout my cancer journey is one of my biggest regrets; I kept far too much of what I felt bottled up inside me. Ironically, my issues with therapy could have been worked out in therapy.

But that day, Dr. Ellis and I had a wonderful phone conversation. For me, therapy is easier over the phone, and you should know that's an option for you if you're uncomfortable seeing a therapist. Towards the end of our conversation, Dr. Ellis and I talked about God. He asked me if I believed in God and to what degree. I am a Reform Jew and always respected God but had never been particularly religious or spiritual. While I found myself praying more since I'd been diagnosed, I hadn't really immersed myself in my belief in God. Dr. Ellis encouraged me to truly seek God's help—if that's what I wanted—because cancer could be an incredible burden to bear myself. So, I did. I talked to God a lot while I healed and really, for the first time in my life, attempted to find spirituality.

I worked towards balancing my fear of death with the belief that God had a plan for me, and however things turned out would be because that's what He, or She, wanted (God might be a woman for all I knew, but I hoped not because I had broken up with a lot of women over the years and felt like a female God might seek retribution).

I told myself that whatever my future held, I would be okay with it. Of course, I didn't really believe that but saying it over and over, like a mantra, made it seem a little truer. To this day it's still hard for me to believe I'll truly be okay with whatever my medical results are, but I know the goal is to feel that way, and I have spent a lot of time working on it. It is way easier said than done, though. I wanted to live then, and I want to live now.

While recovering, I made sure to keep my weight up, because if I went to the doctor and stepped on the scale and lost even a few pounds I would immediately blame cancer. You know, because cancer patients lose weight. Of course, if I gained weight I would make the same assumption and just pick a different reason: a tumor probably weighs a few pounds, and clearly I must have one or two of those inside me.

While dealing with all of this, my girlfriend came down from New York to see me, but by then we merely went through the motions. I couldn't get over her not coming down for my surgeries and not answering the phone before they wheeled me into the operating room. And she resented me for being angry and moody. We mercifully, finally called it quits.

I'm not blaming her for why we fell apart; she's a good woman. There were just too many forces conspiring against us, weighing us down. It broke my heart, but I sought comfort in spirituality, and when I felt my lowest I repeated the mantra, "Give it to God." Those words really started helping me.

During that time, I had the most touching, heartfelt conversation with my father. As I mentioned earlier, while he and I love each other, the one thing we don't do is talk about it. He's taught me to be strong and that's how I have tried to live; even though during this ordeal I was running out of Kleenex.

My dad had a heart attack about 10 years ago and needed triple bypass surgery. He came through it fine, but that experience shook him, and shook all of us. Now, because of cancer I felt like I could relate to his experience, as he could to mine.

While on the couch recovering from surgery and trying to make sense of everything, my dad told me over and over that I would be okay. That all my anxiety would dissipate. It would just take time. He also told me that after his heart attack he reorganized his priorities and devoted much more time to what he wanted to do, rather than what he "had" to do. Those words had a huge effect on me because they allowed me occasional glimpses into what my future might look like; one where I would do more of what I wanted and less of what people wanted me to do.

And we watched a lot of episodes of the show *Vikings*, which made me feel better about my situation. Cancer would have been a typical Tuesday for a Viking. Few of them lived past 30, they rarely bathed, and the women constantly tried to kill the men. After watching that show melanoma didn't seem so bad.

About 10 days into my recuperation, my mother drove me to see family members visiting from New York. I had decided that I wouldn't chase bad news, so I had refused to call the hospital for my results: not even once. It was hard, but I felt good about it.

Then the phone rang. And the call changed my life forever.

The Sylvester Cancer Center's oncology nurse called to remind me that I had an appointment to meet with the oncologist in a few days. I thanked her, but rather than say goodbye, since I had her on the phone anyway, I figured I'd give it a shot. I asked her, "Are my results in yet?"

She told me to hold on while she checked, and I immediately regretted asking.

"Yes," she said, "they're in." And she went silent.

I knew what she was doing: reading my results and deciding if she could tell me or if the doctor had to do it. And if the doctor had to do it, it would be bad. If the cancer spread to any of those lymph nodes, it was probably making its way through my body now and the next PET scan or brain MRI would have different results. I was in the middle of the live-or-die phone call.

More silence on the other end. Followed by mouse clicking and still more silence. I looked at my mom, she looked back at me, neither of us said anything; we prayed as she drove.

And then the nurse spoke. "Okay, Mr. Aizer, normally I would have the doctor call you, but I'll go ahead and give you the results right now."

"Okay," I whispered, my voice barely strong enough to pronounce that one small word.

"Everything looks good," she said, "no spread, everything is negative."

The single greatest sentence in the history of the English language: "Everything is negative." It's ironic how that sentence, with the way it's worded, could be good. I'd never been happier to have "negative" results.

I'm not sure if words can properly describe how I felt at that moment but trust me, if you ever receive that phone call, you'll know. It's like you've been given a second chance at life.

I thanked her and gave my mom the thumbs up, and we both started crying. My mom cried first but watching my mom cry makes me cry every time. This was awesome, but I wasn't convinced. The good news phone call on

Super Bowl Sunday followed by the bad news phone call on Stupor Bowl Monday left me jaded. Before I could celebrate, I needed to be sure this time. I asked the nurse to read me the entire pathology report.

"Lymph nodes one through five, negative for melanoma. Lymph nodes six through eleven, negative for melanoma."

And on it went, every sentence producing tears of joy, until she ran out of lymph nodes. Those three words, negative for melanoma, have been with me ever since that day. I've even saved them on the memo pad in my phone to remind me.

And to this day, thinking about that phone call gets me all choked up. I'm choked up right now as I write this. Freaking cancer, it's turned me into a sap.

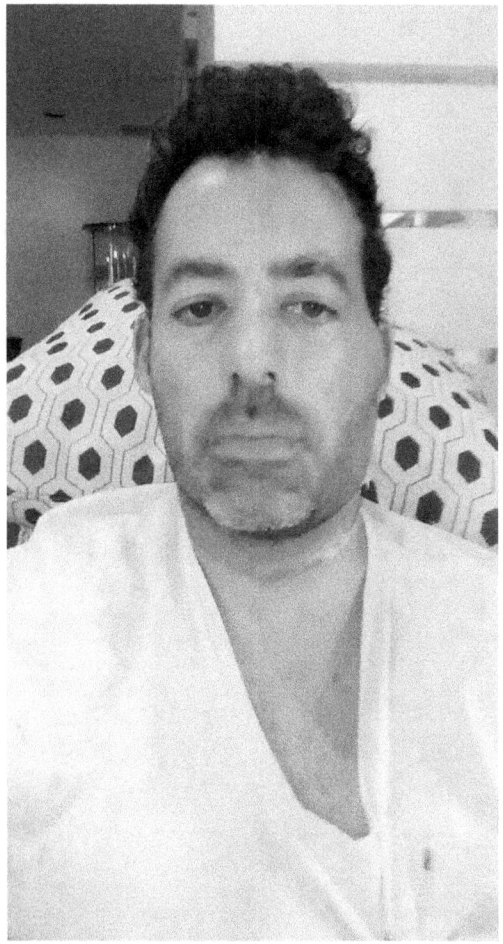

A few days after surgery; it felt even worse than it looked.

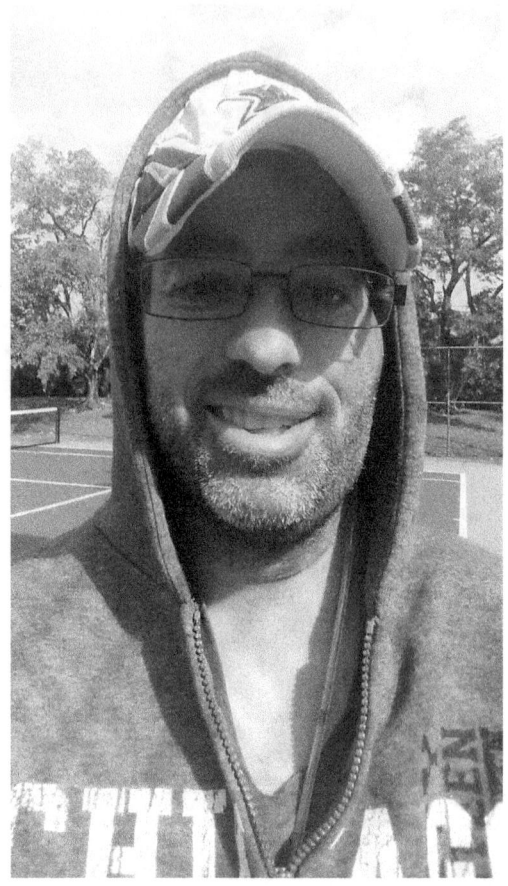

I've got the whole Rocky Balboa crooked smile thing going:
"Yo, Adrienne!"

CHAPTER 11

Potholes On The Road To Recovery

Feeling good about my health, I headed back to the television station. But I had no idea what to expect. My face remained swollen and my eye and lip were droopy, and I didn't know what my coworkers would think of me. It's not like I had a desk job. I was going back to be the "face" of the television station. And let's be honest, my performance would impact my coworkers' financial futures.

For the first bit of good news my key card still worked, so management hadn't decided to fire me without letting me know. In fact, management did quite the opposite. They threw a huge party for me, and everybody said the kindest things. They brought cake, but also herbal tea and organic yogurt. Apparently, my coworkers cared more about my health than I did. My boss even assured me that I had a job at the station for as long as I wanted. I was so blown away by the love everyone showed, I even drank the tea and ate the yogurt.

So now that I had the job, I needed to figure out how to be comfortable doing it again. We rearranged our set, so I'd be sitting to the right of my guests; when I turned to ask them questions the camera would see the right side of my face, not the left. I officially had a "good side." Move over Britney Spears, I was the new diva in town.

I also decided I would let my facial hair grow; not a full Wolf Blitzer beard, but enough scruff to hide some of the swelling and scarring. And when I had to address the camera straight-on I would angle my face ever so subtly. Between all of that and a healthy dose of makeup I was ready for my close-up. Well, not my close-up, but maybe some wide shots.

I thought I had everything figured out and I eagerly resumed my television hosting duties, but before long some viewers sent nasty emails about my swollen face. You might ask why people would do that. It's very simple: they're stupid and they suck.

Rather than wallow in it I chose to embrace it, and I shared my story on camera. That turned out to be the first of many segments I would host about melanoma awareness and prevention, including multiple interviews with my doctors. We got a lot of positive viewer feedback about my story and that's something I am very proud of. In fact, I still regularly discuss melanoma awareness and prevention on camera and on stage. More about that later.

I'd resumed working, the lymph nodes, PET scan, and brain MRI showed no disease, I was developing a taste for herbal tea and my eye and lip were looking closer to normal. Life was awesome. What could possibly stress me out? Well, since this book isn't even at the halfway mark, plenty could still stress me out. For example, the cancer *could* still be in my bloodstream.

One thing about me, I've never been all that good with prosperity. When I'm losing in sports I play great. But give me a lead and I tend to get tight. I start playing not to lose instead of playing to win. Sort of like I expect something to go wrong, and I wait for it to happen. I'm a great opener but not such a great closer.

I am happy to say I'm getting a lot better with this, but back then I always walked on eggshells, waiting for the sky to fall. Instead of basking in the wave of good news, I anticipated the arrival of bad news.

I knew melanoma was one of the more aggressive cancers and that it could come back, even if it seemed gone. I'd heard enough horror stories about that very thing happening, so I lived, every day, waiting for my fortunes to turn. I felt nervous and scared but mostly angry with myself for feeling that way. Meditation didn't help, nor did pep talks. And the fact that I would soon start a treatment program with an oncologist, which would mean frequent doctor visits and more scans, didn't help either. I just couldn't get any distance from melanoma; I'd entered the cancer "protocol" now, and melanoma was omnipresent.

CHAPTER 12

Clinical Trials...
And Tribulations

For my oncologist, I decided on Mount Sinai Medical Center's Dr. Jose Lutzky; a guy so good somebody in the medical community once called him the "Michael Jordan of melanoma care." Can you slam dunk skin cancer? We might be on to a marketing campaign. I must remember to write that down. Wait, I just did.

Dr. Lutzky explained that, based on my stage 3a diagnosis, I had three options: a clinical trial with immunotherapy, a "biologic response modifier" called interferon, or I could choose not to have active treatment and just be closely monitored. The newest FDA-approved melanoma drugs, which were showing some promising results, were only available for patients starting at stage 3b. So, basically, I was diseased enough to have stage 3 cancer, but not quite diseased enough to qualify for the best treatments. I couldn't catch a break!

As for chemotherapy and radiation, they weren't viable options for my disease. Choosing no active treatment was never something I considered, so I could either opt for the clinical trial or interferon. After considerable research, I wanted no part of interferon.

First, interferon hasn't proven to be all that effective stopping melanoma; it only increases your survival rate by roughly 5%. In some people, it's even less than that. And, it beats you to hell. Debilitating migraines, weight loss, hair loss, nausea, depression, anxiety, and numbness in your extremities are just some of many potential side effects. In fact, I had a friend who had taken it years earlier for a different condition, and he made me promise I wouldn't take it. That's how brutal it is. The suggested treatment plan is one year but it's so hard to tolerate, patients rarely stay on it past six months. That coupled with its limited positive results made interferon a no-go for me.

If I chose the clinical trial it would last two years, with injections in my arms and legs every few weeks, and then every few months. The trial was a form of immunotherapy, which is increasingly becoming more and more of a force in the fight against cancer. Rather than chemo which destroys a bunch of cells in your body, immunotherapy stimulates your immune system to work harder and smarter to attack cancer cells. It's sort of like a flu shot, where an inactive flu virus is injected into your body, so the body can develop antibodies to recognize and fight the flu if you get it. As best as I understood it, this trial combined multiple melanoma antigens, which theoretically would help my body seek out and destroy any remaining melanoma cells.

Of course, there was a catch. The trial was 2/3 "active" and 1/3 "placebo," which meant not only did the medical community not know if the drug worked, I wouldn't even know if I was getting the drug in the first place. I could be signing up to get sugar water injections for two years. Again, what does a guy have to do to catch a break around here?

Discouraged, I called my buddy Lee and he told me the "placebo effect" is a real thing, and it has proven to help patients heal. If I proceeded with the trial I needed to convince myself I was getting the medication. That's it. End of story. He was telling me I needed to be optimistic. Had he not met me?

It was a lot to process, and I didn't really like any of my options, but I decided to go with the clinical trial, even though it meant needles, bloodwork, potential side effects and what figured to be a never-ending series of doctor's appointments. Some people probably would have done nothing, and just been monitored, and that would have been there prerogative, but I wouldn't have been able to live with myself if I opted for that path. By taking the trial, I was *actively* choosing to play a role in my care, no matter the outcome. I was proud of that. I felt invested. And I made a promise to myself I would behave as if I was getting the active medication.

Before starting the trial, the remnants of my original mole (yes, they save that stuff) were sent to the lab for mutation testing: not to see if I was a cool mutant like Wolverine, but to see if my melanoma contained any mutations that would make it easier to treat via immunotherapy. The big one was BRAF. If your mole tested BRAF-positive some unique and effective treatment options existed. However, mine tested negative for BRAF as well as all the other testable mutations except for one, NRAS.

When Dr. Lutzky told me this, it bummed me out. I couldn't even tell you what BRAF stood for, but I knew I wanted it. I wanted to be BRAF-positive so badly! He said not to worry and told me it was a good sign the mole tested NRAS-positive, because NRAS responds well to immunotherapy. That was good enough for me and I started the trial embracing my NRAS-positive status even though, to this day, I have no clue what that means. Of course, I could look it up now, but on the off chance I don't like what I read that might set me back and I'm in a good place. So, you can look it up if you'd like.

I dove into the trial, excited to get the process started. But right around the time my trial began, I started fixating on various physical symptoms throughout my body, some real and some imaginary.

CHAPTER 13

You Must Remember This: A Cyst Is Just A Cyst

The saga of my forehead cyst started innocuously enough. I was eating dinner with my friend, Ashley, having a great time and trying to live in the present—an important lesson I had learned in therapy. Ashley and I talked football, relationships, all that nice, normal stuff. I felt like my old self, even if just for a night.

After dinner, we sat outside and continued to shoot the breeze. Not a care in the world. Then a gnat or a mosquito grazed my face. No big deal, it's Florida, stuff like that happens all the time. But as I brushed it off, I felt a bump in the middle of my forehead. It took me precisely 0.03 seconds to associate that bump with cancer, and all hope for a pleasant rest of the evening flew away just like that gnat. It was incredible. Something as inconsequential as a bug had started a tidal wave of panic.

I didn't know what kind of cancer it could be, but surely it was cancer. *Was "forehead cancer" a thing? Maybe bone cancer? Perhaps brain cancer so big that it protruded out of my head? Wait, is my forehead below my brain? Where's my brain again? Are we talking frontal lobe?* I had some sort of metastatic melanoma, that much I knew.

There I was, out of my mind, feverishly poking my forehead outside a P.F. Chang's and asking Ashley to do the same. *How quickly would I die from this? If it was bone cancer or brain cancer, probably soon. Did I have lymph nodes in my forehead?*

A quick WebMD search on my phone indicated that I did not. *Okay then, bone cancer. It was too low to be brain cancer. It had to be bone cancer. After all, melanoma goes to the bones. I read that once.* I was working myself into quite the frenzy.

"Dude," Ashley said. She's from Georgia so she said it with a Southern drawl, which always made me happy… except this time. "It's nothin', relax."

I have heard some variation of, "It's nothing, relax," probably two hundred times since my cancer-related hypochondriasis started. Yet it never resonates. Except maybe when a doctor says it, and a scan confirms it, and a second scan confirms *that* six months later. So, no, I would not be relaxing, dude. Ashley had officially lost me and the pleasure of my company for the evening. There was no going back to talking about football and her beloved Atlanta Falcons.

All I cared about was saying goodbye and getting home as fast as possible, so I could stare at this thing in the mirror, which is exactly what I did. The bump wasn't big; you'd have to squint to see it. To me, though, it looked enormous and cancerous, and I did what any logical person would do: I took out a ruler and measured it. I was going to track this thing every day like meteorologists do an approaching hurricane. The second it got bigger, I would alert the authorities.

But my opinion wasn't enough. The next day, I involved my parents in this madness. I drove an hour to visit them, partly because they're my parents, and I love seeing them, but mostly so they could touch my forehead. I needed other opinions! They poked and prodded; my mom even measured the bump with her ruler just to make sure the numbers aligned. It was like a committee of judges conferring on the length of an Olympic ski jump or something. This was important business.

My sister partook in the insanity too, since she was at the house. There we were, four intelligent humans, standing in the kitchen touching each other's foreheads, checking for lumps and bumps that none of us were even remotely qualified to comprehend.

Over the next few days, I solicited a lot of opinions: some medical professionals, some ordinary folk. No matter how many people told me it was nothing, I wasn't buying it. That is a common theme among hypochondriacs, one I've already mentioned and will do so again. Ninety-nine people could tell us we are fine, but if just one person expresses concern, even if that person is three years old, we're convinced we're in trouble.

I had a physician I play tennis with look at it. He said it was just a cyst. I went to the dentist for a checkup and figured, why not, he has a medical degree, surely, he must know. He too said it was nothing. But two medical opinions weren't enough, so I had my coworkers feel it. That makes total sense, right? Why wouldn't my 23-year-old video editor and my 21-year-old intern be experts on the differences between tumors and cysts? They teach that in journalism school, right?

Anyone with fingers was granted free access to touch my head. It didn't matter how well I knew them; they could proceed like they were kneading dough. This was a full-blown obsession.

Why was I behaving like this? Why was I ignoring common sense and sound medical advice? Why couldn't I move past this irrational, illogical obsession and just be grateful for the day? I think it's because I was so uneasy with all the good news and good test results coming my way, I kept waiting for the other shoe to drop. *Something* had to be wrong, didn't it? After all, this was cancer, and an aggressive cancer at that. And if not the NRAS or the cyst, then something else had to be wrong. What a truly exhausting way to live.

I went to my oncologist, Dr. Lutzky, for my next regularly scheduled checkup. I showed him the cyst, and he wasn't concerned. That should have been it, once and for all.

But it wasn't. I was still concerned. My hypochondriasis, like a cancerous tumor, had grown into paranoia. Clearly everybody was wrong. I was still measuring the damn thing with a ruler every day and, when a ruler wasn't available, I measured it with my fingers.

I went to see my surgeon for a post-surgery checkup. Everything looked good; he seemed pleased with how I was healing. Of course, I had to ask him about the lump. Up until now, nobody had expressed concern, other than me. But if you keep digging around for trouble, and you'll find it.

He wasn't worried, but being extra cautious, he ordered

a blood test to rule out bone cancer and wrote a prescription for a CAT scan of my face to go along with my upcoming neck, chest, stomach, and pelvis CAT scans. There it was, I had succeeded in finding the bad news I desperately sought. And it wasn't even bad news, just a tiny step in that direction. But it validated my concerns and made me feel like less of a lunatic.

Then the blood test and the facial CAT scan came back normal, as did all my other scans, and I felt crazier than ever for wasting so much energy on nothing. Not relieved, not optimistic, just crazy.

Finally, a few days after that, I let it go—and moved onto another malady. We'll get to that soon. But first, as an anecdote to this story, a few months ago, as I scrolled through pictures on my phone, I came upon a picture of me from six years ago, before cancer. And there it was, captured perfectly in the light, the same cyst on my face. Turns out I'd had it the whole damn time. For all I know, I was born with it and just never noticed it before. Boy, did I feel silly, but at least I had a hearty laugh at my own expense.

Learn from me. If you're going through something like this, and you've found a bump or a lump or a mark, check your photo gallery before having a nervous breakdown. It may have been there since birth.

CHAPTER 14

Here's Mud In Your Sty

As we all know, stress wreaks havoc on your body and can create all sorts of ailments, real and perceived. In my case, it did a little bit of both. One such ailment was a sty in my right eye, or as I called it: "ocular melanoma."

Actually, I didn't know if it was ocular melanoma or mucosa melanoma, but I had a strong feeling it was one of those two melanomas. I mean, I knew nothing about either of those things, other than they existed; they involved your eye, and could both kill you. And I found plenty of terrifying articles on the internet to confirm my misguided suspicions.

Maybe it was just a sty. I'd never had a sty before. Who gets sties? Oh wait, apparently a lot of people do. They're common. And they look exactly like what I have. They can be caused by stress, and I'm unbelievably stressed out, so that fits.

Nah, I'm going with cancer.

I remember the morning I woke up with it. If you've had one, you know how painful they are; if you haven't, trust me, they hurt. It's basically a bump that forms in your eyelid due to a blocked gland. It's a constant throbbing pain. And they don't look so fantastic, either—especially when you're on television.

Not only was the left side of my face scarred and still healing from the surgery, and my left eye still sagged a bit, but now I had a bump underneath my right eye. Both sides of my face were disfigured. There were no flattering camera angles left anymore, unless we shot my show in the dark.

I had a shoot that afternoon, so I tried to cover the sty with makeup. That just made things worse. For every layer of makeup I applied over the sty, I applied an equal amount over the rest of my face. After the fifth layer, there was so much makeup caked on me I looked like the sadistic doll Chucky from *Child's Play*. I was destined for a career on the Syfy channel. Of course, if the melanoma had spread to my eye, it was going to be a short career. There might not even be a second season.

I called my ophthalmologist, Dr. Norman Kline, and he suggested applying warm compresses to my face. It didn't work. After wondering if the compresses weren't warm enough, I made them hotter—and I burned my face. I was falling apart by the second. My sty hurt, my face was burnt, I was a ticking time bomb mentally, and my arm was exhausted from holding a towel to my face for 15 minutes. On the plus side, it is hard to Google ocular melanoma with only one free arm and one good eye. I had that going for me.

After a few days, the sty stopped hurting. Now it was just an eye sore...literally. But it wasn't going away, and sties were supposed to go away. Why wasn't it going away? Clearly because it wasn't a sty at all; it was cancer; and cancer doesn't go away. That was the logical conclusion.

But let's think about this for a minute. I had just had a CAT scan on my face, plus blood tests per my clinical trial protocol, plus, as it turned out, an eye exam a few months ago. All of those were clean. I was fine. This was nothing, said 98% of the world's rationally thinking population. The other irrational 2%, me included, would choose to see this completely full glass as mostly empty.

After a few more days of scorching hot compresses that did nothing, I resolved to get this sucker removed. As it turns out, the only thing more painful than a sty is having a sty removed. But Dr. Kline took good care of me, and it was a pretty simple process. Unfortunately, apparently after having a sty you are more prone to having another one. Hasn't happened yet, but that's something to look forward to.

Incidentally, I have also experienced the occasional "eye floater," when you see spots floating across your field of vision. Like sties, they are apparently normal and no cause for concern. I had forgotten about them until just now when I noticed a few of them. It could be because I've been staring at this computer for a few hours, or because I've been wearing the same lenses for a few weeks, or because of a massive brain tumor. It's too tough to tell at this point.

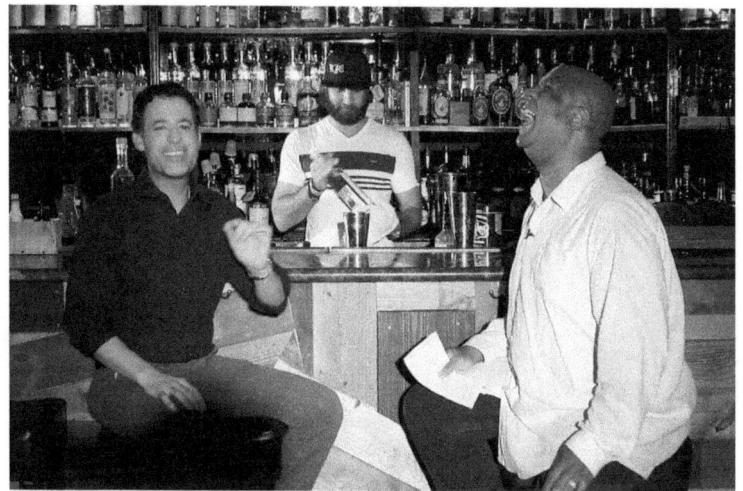

Even my friend Rod Hagwood is laughing at all my makeup.

CHAPTER 15

Signs From God

Right around the sty saga, still just a few months after my cancer diagnosis, I started to play a little game with myself. Not a fun game like, "Are those people dating or related?" Nope, this game was called "Signs from God," and it offered further proof I was losing my mind. Here's how you play:

At least 10 times a day I asked for a sign from Above to let me know if I was cancer-free or if the cancer was spreading throughout my body. Basically, my way of finding out if I was dying. To be clear, this in no way is what my therapist meant when he suggested I get closer to God but, while that was a work in progress, this guaranteed me immediate answers.

For example, I would say, "Okay God, if I know the next song on the radio, my cancer is gone." Because apparently God moonlights as a radio disc jockey. Then I would turn on the radio; if I knew the song I had a clean bill of health, but if I didn't, I was a dead man walking. If I turned on the radio and heard a commercial, I really wasn't sure what to think—except, as a pessimist, since I didn't know all the words to the commercial, I took that as a bad sign.

Here are some more examples of things that would indicate I had cancer: coins that landed on tails, if my brother called me David instead of Dave, if my station's television ratings were bad, if the forecast called for rain, if the bistro ran out of goat cheese, if my parents' garage door opened on the first try (it had a tendency to stick), if I won in tennis, if I lost in tennis, and so on. It all made sense to me, and I totally bought into it. To me, this was way more scientific than actual science.

I'm not going to lie: I didn't always play fairly. You could say I was the Bill Belichick of this game. I would often play "Signs from God" with the deck stacked in my favor. Like, if I could open the refrigerator with three fingers, no cancer. Of course, I could do that; I'm not a five-year-old. Or if I could do a one-minute plank, that meant no cancer. I typically *could* manage that, and even if I struggled, I'd just cheat a little on my form. Nobody was watching—except God. God is always watching.

In that case, would the wager be nullified because God saw me cheat? If he saw me cheat, why did he let me do the plank in the first place? It's a complicated game.

I wish I could say that now, over four years after my original diagnosis, I have stopped playing this game. I really wish I could say that because, man, does this make me sound mentally unbalanced. But, alas, I still play it from time to time. Just played it this morning based on the amount of milk I had left for my coffee. Good news: I did indeed have enough for a cup, so, no cancer. But, I didn't have enough for a second cup, so I'm not sure where that leaves me.

CHAPTER 16

Rising Above My Fears

With all the lows I was experiencing, it was time for a much-needed high. And since we've established I'm way too paranoid for marijuana, I was going to have to get my high from heights. So, I had the bright idea that it would be fun to rappel down a 30-story building. Actually, a marketing executive had the bright idea, but it was for charity, a cancer charity no less, so I couldn't turn that down.

Gilda's Club is an organization named in honor of the late comedienne and *Saturday Night Live* alum Gilda Radner, who died of ovarian cancer. It's a support group for everyone living with cancer: not just patients, but their friends, family, and caregivers. They have an office in South Florida and, in spring 2015, they raised awareness by inviting members of the local media to scale down the 110 Tower—the tallest building in Ft. Lauderdale.

For all the fears I have, surprisingly, fear of heights is not one of them. In fact, I've been skydiving and it's among the most thrilling things I've done. While I was a tiny bit nervous about rappelling, it felt like a way to take back some control over my life and give cancer the finger—even if it was just for one afternoon.

So, I went for it. My television station brought a camera crew to film me going "Over the Edge" for charity. It started out fine; I had no trouble standing on the building's roof, going through the safety protocol. It all sounded exciting and pretty simple. I'd be attached to a harness and walk my way down the building, backwards. No problem at all. I could do that. Then it was my turn to go and suddenly it didn't feel so exciting anymore.

I made my way to the edge of the building, 410 feet off the ground. Next, I had to turn around, face backwards and place my feet on the edge of the building. Say, what? I must have missed that part in the instruction manual! But, I managed to do it and planted my toes while my heels dangled in the wind. My legs turned to jelly.

One task remained before launch: I needed to jump backwards to gain enough momentum; simply falling backwards wouldn't cut it. I tried to jump; I really did— multiple times. But while my mind said, "jump," my body said, "screw you." I stood there frozen, overcome with terror. Life hit me with another challenge, and once again

I couldn't handle it. I wasn't strong enough to deal with cancer, and I wasn't strong enough to jump. I felt a myriad of emotions with self-loathing at the top of the list.

Then, as all hope seemed lost, I looked at my producer, Bianca, who was videotaping me, and she said, "You got this." Bianca is as sweet as they come and a very good friend, but she can also be rather impatient. So, while I'm assuming her encouraging words came from a place of love, there's a chance she'd grown tired of waiting for me to jump and just wanted me to do it already. We were on a deadline, after all. Still, I'm choosing to believe it was the more nurturing of the two options.

I jumped, throwing caution, and my body, to the wind. And it was awesome! I was Spiderman; bouncing off the building, descending story by story, feeling unstoppable. Nothing could touch me, not even cancer. I would live the rest of my life like this! I would take chances, I would laugh in the face of danger, I would be bold. I would…uh oh…I was stuck.

It's not enough to jump off the building and then jump from floor to floor; you must do all that at a certain pace. If you jump too quickly or too slowly the rope gets stuck and you can't move. And that, my friends, is what happened to me; I hung there, suspended mid-air, roughly 300 feet off the ground.

I full-on panicked. Catastrophic feelings rushed to the surface, and I worried I'd be stuck there for hours waiting on a fireman to rescue me. Since there were other news personalities waiting to rappel, with their camera operators standing by, I feared the entire ordeal would end up on all the local newscasts—with me in the arms of some buff firefighter, like a damsel in distress. And for some reason I pictured him shirtless, his perfect abs glistening while I held on to him for dear life. That would have been epically humiliating. But, after a few moments, my imagination took a timeout and those feelings subsided, and I just started laughing.

My fear turned to amusement. I mean, at this point, what the hell else could go wrong? It was like cancer tried to give me the middle finger right back, but I wouldn't have it. I soaked it all in and looked down at the ground below and at the city all around me. It was incredible. I felt closer to God, literally and figuratively, at that moment than I had been in a long time, and I believe he made the rope get stuck, so I could take a minute and appreciate being alive. After months of consistent, unyielding terror, finally a moment where I could enjoy the beauty of life.

I lived in that moment, fully present. The rope eventually became unstuck, I made my way down the building and celebrated life with handshakes, hugs and a cold beer.

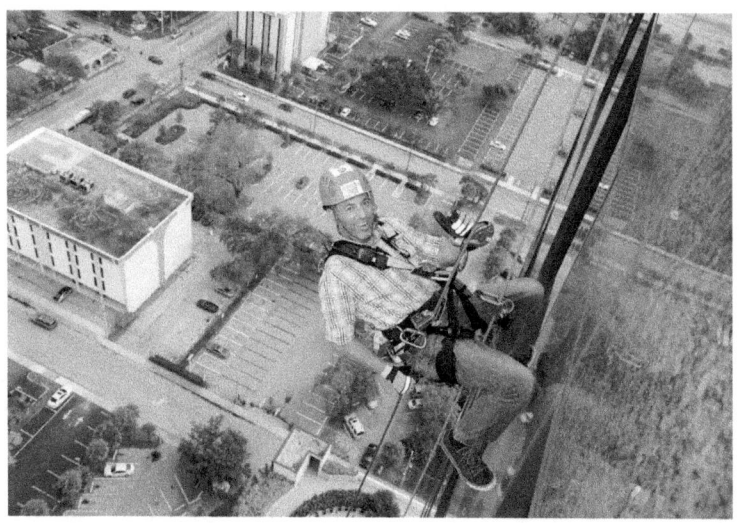

I'm enjoying the view, and the blessings of life, a few hundred feet in the air.

CHAPTER 17

Single And Ready To (Awkwardly) Mingle

Bolstered by my newfound appreciation for life I decided to start putting myself "out there." I wasn't sure I was ready to fall in love with somebody and spend our Saturdays buying monogrammed towels, but I was definitely on board with some human companionship.

I dipped my toe into the dating pool, but it was like I had forgotten how to swim. I'd always been rather good at talking to women, but now I didn't how, or when, to bring up cancer. I wasn't sure what the protocol was for when to bring up the, "I just had melanoma and, you know, it could come back and kill me" conversation. That's not in the handbook.

My friends and family said I didn't have to mention anything right away, certainly not on the first date. Let it come up on its own; no need to lead with it. So, naturally,

I mentioned it right away, five minutes into date one, every single time.

This happened in part because of my self-consciousness about my scars and the residual swelling, and partly because melanoma was all I'd talked about for months and I didn't know how to have a conversation without bringing it up.

I figured, screw it, if I was going to talk about it I might as well use it to my advantage. After all I had survived one of the most aggressive cancers out there. The ladies didn't have to know I was rubbing the cyst on my head 20 times a day and googling ocular melanoma every five minutes. No, I was a warrior; I kicked cancer's ass AND rappelled down a building. And check out my scars. Damn, I'm sexy.

I made the conversation relatable, no matter who I dated. On a date with a black woman, I'd say, "Bob Marley died of melanoma. It can happen to anyone." When I took a Jewish girl out, it would be, "My dad is Israeli with dark skin. I can't believe I got melanoma." And if I had the pleasure of an Irish girl's company, particularly one with red hair and freckles, I'd say, "You should definitely go to a dermatologist. You need to be careful." I became the United Nations of melanoma one-liners, even if some of the lines weren't very smooth.

I would have conversations at bars with women I didn't know and wait for them to bring up the beach (South Floridians almost always talk about the beach). That would launch me straight into my tale of heroism. And if they wouldn't bring up the beach, I would. And when they eventually asked me if I liked the beach I would say, "Well I have skin cancer, so I don't really go to the beach." And then they'd give me a hug.

Cancer became my go-to pick up line. And if you really apply yourself, it can be yours as well.

But, because I'm an over-thinker, I alternated between taking dating seriously (or at least quasi-seriously) and adopting the attitude of, "Screw it, life is short and who knows what tomorrow holds so I'm just going to spend crazy amounts of money on really hot women and fly them places because it's fun."

Sadly, I have made so many bad decisions in my dating life, pre and post-cancer that if I mentioned them all, I would run out of nouns, verbs and adjectives. Like I always said, it took real skill to be 40 and never married. That's not easy to do! So, I'll just share one dating story (a post-cancer story) to give you a good idea as to what you're dealing with here.

I went on six or seven dates with a woman who was, without question, a horrible choice for me as a mate. We

had nothing in common, she was just getting out of a relationship, and she was seriously considering leaving South
Florida. Not exactly soulmate material, but she looked
great in jeans.

So, with life being short and precious, and money just
being an object, and her having a phenomenal body, I
decided to fly her cross country for a long weekend with
me. Mind you in our six or seven dates we hadn't even
kissed—not once, not even by accident. But hey, my cancer
could come back at any point, so screw it.

I totally understand how people who get diagnosed
with cancer spend all their money on cars and trips and
material stuff. Money doesn't matter too much at that point.
If you've been diagnosed, spend your money, you've earned
it; just don't take someone on vacation who is apparently
allergic to kissing you. And if there's a pretty good chance
you're going to live, maybe don't spend all your money
because, you know, you'll need it when you're alive and stuff.

I will spare you the self-deprecating and painfully
awkward details of that weekend and cut to the end of the
story. We didn't kiss, we barely hugged, and we rubbed
shoulders once but that was by accident on a crowded
sidewalk. I didn't even ask her to feel my armpit lymph
nodes or touch my cyst, so clearly there was no intimacy

there. By the end of the weekend we hardly spoke, and I can talk to anyone. I even got us on an earlier flight just to end the trip as soon as possible, and on the flight home I put my headphones on (but didn't listen to anything) to rule out any chance of a potential conversation. I was out a few thousand dollars and three days of my life.

That weekend proved to be a dating turning point. I decided not to chase love, and to let it come to me. I had enough other stuff to deal with so relationships took a back seat for a while. But with a void of meaningful companionship outside of my family, I needed something to fill me with purpose. And I found that purpose in advocacy.

CHAPTER 18

A Perfect Day For A 5K

In October 2015, almost a year after diagnosis, I was itching to positively impact the world. I had become determined to start using my cancer diagnosis to educate, inform, and inspire others. Truth be told, although I was feeling better, I still had my share of dark days and bouts with anxiety. I spent part of every day waiting for my cancer to come back and couldn't say with any certainty how much longer I'd be alive. But whether I had two years on this planet or 50, I had to be a force for good, just like JoAnna had been for me.

Sure, I had shared my story on television, and I was blessed to have done so, but I hadn't been able to connect with many people in person. That included sun-worshippers putting themselves at risk, and people who, in one way or another, had already been touched by melanoma.

I reached out to the Melanoma Research Foundation, one of the premiere melanoma organizations in the country, and began what would become a beautiful relationship that continues today. On November 1st of that year the MRF was scheduled to hold its "Miles for Melanoma" 5K on Key Biscayne, about an hour south of Ft. Lauderdale. They asked me to emcee the event and I was beyond honored to do so.

The night before the 5K I was nervous. The next day I would meet hundreds of people who had lost loved ones to the disease or were suffering from it themselves. I kept thinking of all the sad stories I might hear. Whereas JoAnna's story of survival brought me hope, stories of death and sickness could send me spiraling.

Amazingly, the exact opposite happened. I noticed an incredible sense of community from the moment I arrived, and I knew nobody would let me feel sorry for myself. After I shared my story to the group before the start of the race, people came over to me, one after another, and hugged me. People I had never met before kept telling me I would be all right and that I should live every moment to its fullest and be grateful for the day. Boy did I feel grateful for that day. It was the first time since my cancer diagnosis that I'd been around a community of people just like me.

And we all wore *a lot* of sunscreen.

Your family and your doctors can fill you with love, well-wishes and hope, but when fellow cancer warriors do it, it's truly incredible. That remains one of the best days of my life. And I recommend, if you do have cancer, to meet other survivors. I think a 5K is a great place to do it. People are generally very positive there. I've never been to a support group, so I can't really speak about it, but a few friends have told me those groups can be quite sad and death is frequently discussed. Personally, I wouldn't go down that road because a positive mental outlook is so important in this process. But it might be worth a try. Just know, whatever route you choose, there is strength in numbers.

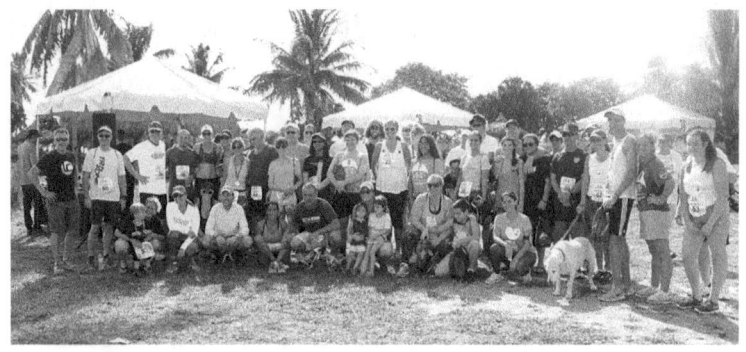

The Miles for Melanoma 5K: surrounded by a community of melanoma warriors.

CHAPTER 19

"Dude, Why Is Your Face Sweating?"

By December 2015, I was feeling much better physically and still coming off the high from the 5K. It had been about nine months since my second surgery and I'd regained my strength, my clinical trials were painless, and I was getting in really good shape. The cancer hadn't returned and, even though I worried about it daily, nothing specific indicated it would. The scars had faded a bit, the swelling was gone, and even though my left eye sagged a little and I had some facial asymmetry, there was nothing physical to suggest I had been through hell. So naturally, something bad had to happen: I got the "face sweats."

During my second surgery the surgeon had removed my parotid gland. It had to come out because microscopic cancer existed right around it. Doctors explained to me that as a side effect I might experience sweat on the side of my face when I ate, due to something called Frey's Syndrome. Here's the medical explanation: typically, during surgical trauma to the parotid gland the auriculotemporal nerve is injured. When the nerve heals it reattaches to sweat glands instead of the salivary gland, because the parotid isn't there anymore. That means, instead of salivating when I ate, I would sweat.

It sounded horrible, but at the time I didn't care. I had enough other stuff on my plate, if you will. And it didn't happen, so I forgot about it. But right around Christmas, at a holiday dinner party, it indeed began. My very own Christmas miracle: a sweaty face for all to enjoy. God bless us, everyone.

There I was, celebrating the birth of Jesus, or as us Jews call it, a day we get off from work, eating Italian food when, without warning, the left side of my face got wet. I assumed it was from my drink, so I wiped it. A few bites later, wet face again. *Was I drunk? Had I forgotten how to eat?* I wiped it, took another bite, and it came back, over and over again. Before long it dawned on me: that sweaty face thing the doctors warned me about is here. That's just freaking great!

Unfortunately, that little peculiarity has not faded with time. At pretty much every meal since then I have

"DUDE, WHY IS YOUR FACE SWEATING?"

experienced the same unfortunate occurrence: taking a bite, sweating, and wiping my face, repeatedly. The constant napkin wiping makes me seem like quite the messy eater. The sweat isn't even near my mouth, so it must look ridiculous to my dining companions. And it's not like certain foods trigger it more than others, so I can find a "safe zone." Indian food, Greek food, a turkey sandwich, even a piece of gum…they're all equal offenders.

Oh, and it's not just from eating; sweating can also appear when I see, dream, think about, or even talk about food. Anything that gets the blood, or in this case, sweat, percolating. If I were a sleepwalker I could accomplish all those things simultaneously.

This made me very self-conscious for a while, but as I've progressed I've learned not to let it bother me so much. After all, everybody has "stuff." In fact, like my scars, it's become a reason for me to engage someone in a conversation about my melanoma.

People sometimes ask about my scars and when I tell them what happened, and we spend time talking about melanoma, they say things like, "You should come up with a cool story, like a shark attacked you or something." And I tell them, the truth is even cooler. These are my battle scars and every time I look at them in the mirror, or every time my face sweats from eating, I'm reminded about my cancer journey. And I'm good with that. I'm proud of my scars.

That said, it would be great to eat a steak without a box of napkins.

CHAPTER 20

Between A Hard Rock And A Hard Place

The calendar turned to 2016 marking the one-year anniversary of my initial diagnosis. All things considered, I was doing all right. I mean, I was a neurotic mess with a sweaty left side of my face, but there was plenty of good news and positive momentum and I was learning to celebrate that stuff. I was cancer-free and in the mood to party.

In early January my family and I embarked on a week-long vacation to the beautiful Hard Rock Resort in Punta Cana, Dominican Republic. All signs pointed to this being a week in paradise.

The hotel, the weather, and the scenery were magnificent. The trip felt like the perfect way to start off 2016 after a mostly crappy 2015. Granted I had a brain MRI scheduled for the week after my vacation, so that was on my mind, but I was determined not to think about any of that stuff for a week. Heck, I even planned to lie out on the beach. With sunscreen, long sleeves and a hat, but still, I would lie out.

Just like that movie where Stella got her groove back on vacation—I would soon get mine. But my tropical good-time buzz lasted approximately one day.

The morning of day two I woke up in my luxurious king-sized bed with a smile on my face and not a care in the world. The sun was shining and there was tennis to play; the day was mine. Then I saw the blood.

Dried blood stained my bed sheet, right near my neck. How could this be and where did it come from? *Did I bleed during the night? Did I have another melanoma?*

One warning sign of melanomas is that they bleed. I didn't know that the first time and ignored two separate occasions of dried blood on my pillow. Had I known, I might have been able to do something about it sooner. I wouldn't make the same mistake twice.

But how could I have another melanoma? I go to the dermatologist every three months, and the last time I went he didn't see anything suspicious. *Could this really be happening again?*

Straight out of *Dexter*, I did a forensic crime-scene reen-actment. I rolled around the bed, under the sheets, trying to replicate all the possible angles where my body could have left this patch of blood. It was a good amount of blood and it was fully dry, which seemed odd because if this much blood seeped out of me some of it should have still been wet, but still I panicked.

Where was this new mole? Did I bleed from my nose or even my mouth? And for the love of God, why now? I was on vacation!

So, I did what any 41-year-old man on vacation without a girlfriend would do. I called my mom for help. Don't get me wrong, I would have rather asked my girlfriend or my wife but, as I didn't have either of those, mom was next on the list.

She came to my room and helped me process my crime-scene data analysis. We didn't touch the blood; we had boundaries. We just got right up close to it, examined it, and reached the conclusion that if that much blood had left my body overnight there would be a scratch or some other discernible mark on me. And since we didn't see blood on me, or any funky-looking moles, our final report was that the blood wasn't mine. Which made me happy until I realized what that meant: I slept under a sheet all night with somebody else's dried blood on it.

Gross.

I marched straight down to the concierge and let him have it. I hit him with a one-two punch of germ phobia and hypochondriasis and closed with a fury of cancer—a verbal beat down the likes of which had never been seen at the Hard Rock. In fact, I'm guessing they still refer to me as that "loco gringo."

Granted, the concierge didn't speak English so much of the message might have been lost in translation. But I feel like my flailing arms told the story. My crisis made its way up the chain of command, and after some back and forth guess who got a free deluxe massage: this guy. At that point I clearly needed a massage. Sadly, though, the vacation had just begun, and things would get worse.

Of all the embarrassing things I have mentioned, and will mention, in this book the one I'm about to share is the most embarrassing. It's so embarrassing I debated leaving it out of the book entirely. But if it in some small way it makes even one of you feel better about yourself then it's worth it, I suppose…even though it probably isn't.

Let's start with this. I am color-blind. Not all the way color-blind where I only see black and white, but moderately color-blind where certain colors and shades give me fits. Add that to the list of my quirks.

Back in college, I rushed the fraternity Sigma Alpha Mu

and accepted a bid from them in large part because their colors were navy blue and white, and navy blue was my favorite color. The day I accepted their bid and became a pledge I bought one of their t-shirts, to proudly wear around campus. About five minutes after that a friend asked me why I had joined a purple fraternity. I insisted my shirt was blue, he confirmed it was purple, and that ended that discussion.

Two of the colors that confuse me the most are red and brown, a problem which would soon bite me in the butt. A few hours after the bloody sheet episode I went to the bathroom, and as I finished wiping myself I noticed some blood on the toilet paper. More blood! This day felt like the prom scene from *Carrie*.

At least it looked like blood. Was it red or brown? I squinted but couldn't tell for sure. I brought the toilet paper in for a closer look but still didn't know. So, and here comes the worst part, I smelled it. Yep, I stood in my hotel room, over the toilet, smelling my soiled toilet paper to determine it was feces or blood. The second day of my trip to paradise, and this was how I was spending my morning.

Please know I haven't done any of this since that trip. It's not a fetish of mine. Now that we've gotten that out of the way, back to the story.

I was pretty sure it indeed was blood. Back to WebMD

I went. Hemorrhoids seemed to be a possible, if not probable, conclusion. I ventured over to the mirror and I will spare you what happened next but suffice it to say I gave myself a thorough exam, which isn't easy to do at that angle, by the way.

Not finding anything, my thoughts turned to colon cancer. I spent a good part of the next couple of days eating excessively and drinking lots of coffee to speed up my internal plumbing, so I could get a better sample size. I excused myself from lunches, dinners, and swimming pool hangouts for multiple trips to the restroom, each one, turning into a toilet paper examination.

In the end, pun very much intended, I'm pretty sure what I saw on the morning of day two was not blood, just good old-fashioned poop, but by day four there indeed was some bleeding. Not because of cancer, mind you; because of the hotel's sandpaper-like toilet paper and the frequency and aggressiveness with which I was applying it.

That might have been hard for you all to read, but I assure you it was no picnic to relive. In terms of embarrassment, here's hoping I just hit rock bottom, or Hard Rock bottom as it were.

One final episode of vacation misfortune was still to come. I mentioned earlier I had a brain MRI set for when I returned to Florida. As much as I tried not to think about it, I couldn't help it, it was on my mind—which I believe is normal, by the way. How can you not think about an impending brain exam? I became hyper-aware of everything going on in my head, like the occasional ringing in my ears when I would lie down. It's called tinnitus and it's common, and for all I know it had been there for years, but now that I was focused on it the ringing sounded like a concert in my eardrums. After a night or two of obsessing about it, I went back to my favorite website WebMD for info and, believe it or not, got some good news. It seems ringing in both ears is typically not indicative of a brain tumor whereas ringing in one ear may be a bit more of a problem. And since my tinnitus was in stereo I could move on from it.

That led me right into the coup-de-grace of brain-related meltdowns: what I call the "burnt toast episode." Somewhere tucked deep in the recesses of my mind I had stored a nugget I had once heard about brain cancer. I couldn't place who told me, or if I had seen it in a movie, but I remembered somebody describing the smell of imaginary burnt toast as a symptom of a brain tumor.

Around night five of my week-long vacation from hell I awoke in the middle of the night smelling something burning. Something was on fire, but I had no idea what, or where it was. It wasn't in the room, which was obviously a good sign because, you know, I would have died. I stepped onto the balcony and didn't see any smoke, so the fire didn't seem to be coming from outside either. This was *not* a good sign because it left only one place the smell could be coming from: my brain tumor. I washed my face, as if that might help. It didn't. I held my nose for a few seconds as if to reset my smell mechanism. That didn't help either. I still smelled smoke and was out of ideas. This was it: the brain tumor I knew would come for me.

Panicked, I called the front desk to see if there indeed was a fire. Nobody answered. Maybe all the employees evacuated and chose not to tell me. Maybe one of them said, "The building is on fire, we must leave! Call all the guests!" And another one said, "I already did, except for the guy who bitched about his sheets! Let him burn." And, then they both laughed. That seemed like a stretch but I wasn't thinking clearly.

I quickly dressed. It was a long walk to the front desk as my room was in a building far from the main lobby. But I needed to walk; in part to ask about the fire and in part to say my last goodbyes and make my peace with the Lord. I was going to die via blaze or tumor. The end was near, one way or another. So, I headed to the lobby at 4 a.m., all the while smelling smoke and sniffing around like a Basset Hound. Upon reaching the lobby the smell of smoke overwhelmed me. Nobody else seemed bothered, further proof of my impending demise.

Before I could say anything, the concierge (a different one than the bloody sheet guy), greeted me with, "Good evening, sir, we apologize for the smell of smoke. There was a brush fire, but it is under control."

"Oh," I said, "thanks." And just like that, I walked back to my room: simultaneously relieved and furious with myself. I sat on the bed and laughed, a lot.

The vacation, which my family so lovingly organized in large part for me, had become a disaster due to one imagined crisis after another. What happened to the guy who rappelled down the building? Where's the warrior who bonded with fellow melanoma survivors at the 5K? All the work I put in to get to this place of optimism was disintegrating. I needed to get a handle on this situation. This had to stop immediately.

I got into the room, made a deal to be nicer to myself, and went to sleep. And the next morning I celebrated my perfect health with a real piece of toast and enjoyed the rest of my time in Punta Cana.

CHAPTER 21

My Neck, My Back, My Panic Attack

As it turned out I salvaged my vacation, and I came back from Punta Cana rejuvenated, refreshed, and slightly tan, which for me was a huge deal. Don't get me wrong I wore sunscreen the whole time, but still managed to get some color. That initially made me uneasy, but I had been very conscientious about staying out of the sun, so I made my peace with it and figured what's meant to be will be. It might not sound like much, but I had made an active choice to not worry about something and for that I gave myself credit.

One of the problems the melanoma community struggles with is that people inherently look better when they're tan so by asking them to stay out of the sun you're essentially asking them to not look their best. It's an uphill battle. Therefore, melanoma organizations specifically don't ask people to shy away from the sun. Their message is not less sun; it's more sun safety. They want people to enjoy the sun, but do so responsibly, rather than be afraid of it. I've always found that interesting.

Anyway, my brain MRI came back clean, giving me reason to celebrate. The ringing in my ears soon went away, and I never smelled burnt toast again. The year 2016 did in fact start way better than 2015. The next couple of months were, more or less, uneventful. I played a ton of tennis, laughed a lot, and felt truly blessed to be alive. I ate better, meditated, and spent less and less time worrying about symptoms.

To feel even more relaxed, I decided to start getting massages every month. After all, I had enjoyed my complimentary Hard Rock massage so much, how could it not be a great idea to get more of them? And that, my friends, is where it all fell apart yet again. Halfway into my first massage since Hard Rock, I became convinced I had cancer in my back and my neck.

Speaking of back and neck, it was quite the pain in the neck that my hypochondriasis was back. I can't speak for other cancer patients, but I know the constant back and forth between mental health and mental anguish was the hardest part for me. Much harder than any physical pain I felt. Every time I thought I had it beat, something would happen, and I would revert to crisis mode. I know some of these stories are funny, but mostly they were exhausting and crippling and really sad. I wish, upon my retelling of these stories, that I had committed to consistent psychotherapy much earlier than I ultimately did.

Back to my back, and the lipoma I've had for probably 20 years. A lipoma, if you don't know, is a harmless fatty lump between skin and muscle that is almost always non-cancerous and therefore not a cause for concern. I have one right in the middle of my back, next to my spine. It's never changed size, and it's never bothered me at all, but during the massage the therapist ran her hand over it and, although she didn't say anything, I could tell she was curious about it. Surely there must be something wrong. I began jumping to conclusions.

But she had more damage to inflict upon my fragile psyche. The massage therapist soon moved to the left side of my neck, an area that's perpetually sore from the surgeries and the reconstruction and where numbness and tingling come and go at will. It will probably never feel quite like it used to, but I rarely notice it. However, this time, as she pressed down on my neck, I felt the pronounced lump around my scar.

I was in a room with dim lighting, soft music, and eucalyptus, supposed to be getting my Zen on, yet counting the minutes until this woman would get her hands off me so I could get dressed, leave, go home, and stare at my back and neck in the mirror. I finished the massage in a far more stressful state than I had started it. Don't worry, I still tipped her.

For the next couple of weeks, I examined my neck and back nonstop. I examined them mostly separately, but occasionally at the same time.

The problem is that touching my lipoma proved to be hard because it sat on the middle of my back. Measuring it proved to be next to impossible. Try touching the middle of your back. Now try measuring part of it with your fingers. Not very easy, is it? I ended up cutting my back with my fingernails from the incessant probing. After a while, I had to give up because the awkward arm movement was killing my shoulder.

"How did you tear your rotator cuff?"

" Measuring my lipoma."

"Oh, okay. Cool story. Stay away from my kids."

So, like I did with the cyst on my head, I enlisted family members to help me measure it, which meant walking around my parents' house lifting my shirt, or taking it off entirely, and asking my mom, dad and sister to touch my back. I swear we're normal. Well, they are.

Eventually I tired of this and moved past it when enough people told me to stop, allowing me to focus on the lump in my neck.

You may ask, what specifically was I looking for? No idea. For starters, I had been getting regular neck scans every three months, so I shouldn't have been the least bit concerned about cancer. Plus, in the second operation my surgeon removed pretty much everything from that side of my neck so, unless I magically regrew lymph nodes, there really couldn't be anything in there to cause me harm.

However, me being me, I reasoned that because there had been so much reconstruction in that area perhaps something might have been missed in a CAT scan. So, I called my radiologist with one hand, while pressing down on my neck with the other. He reassured me it was highly unlikely I had anything to worry about. Next, I called my buddy Lee, the head and neck surgeon. He also told me not to worry and, without benefit of looking at it or feeling it, seemed sure it was scar tissue.

"But what if they missed a few lymph nodes during the surgery and those had become infected?" I asked.

"No chance," he said.

Those two opinions should have been enough, and they were, for a few hours.

Later that day I was back at square one, rubbing my neck like a fool and not trusting two doctors whom I hold in the highest esteem. This seems like a good time to mention that I was *already* rubbing my face every single day for 15 minutes for an entirely different reason. According to my plastic surgeon, rubbing the swollen surgical areas in a downward motion would reduce the buildup of post-surgical lymphatic fluid and make my face more symmetrical, closer to how it looked before.

So even though I was one-year post surgery, and probably past the point of my face changing its shape anymore, I still rubbed my face a few times a day. And now, I added my neck to the routine. Every day at work, in the car, on the couch, in a meeting, wherever...I was the guy rubbing his face and neck. Whether I was alone or around people, it didn't matter. It became second nature. My friends and colleagues would laugh at me, but how else could I get my face back to normal while simultaneously checking for neck tumors.

CHAPTER 22

Liver, Foot, And Thigh, Oh My!

My body rubbing soon expanded past my face and neck. I had started down a dark road and that road would take me to my liver and thighs before finally stopping at my feet. The liver is a hot spot for melanoma spread, and now that my hypochondriasis was supercharged once again, it didn't take long for me to settle on that spot as my cancer's next possible target.

I'd been getting stomachaches, probably from the anxiety caused by obsessing about my neck and back, and after a few days in a row I felt certain the cancer had spread to my liver. Never mind I didn't exactly know how to find my liver, how to check it, or what to check for; I started poking the right side of my stomach repeatedly. This, predictably, caused it to hurt, which, predictably, caused more fear that I had liver disease. On it went with me once again discounting, if not blatantly ignoring, my previous negative scans and the counsel of my very smart physicians.

I remember one work meeting, in particular. My team sat around discussing our television production schedule for the week. I tend to zone out in these meetings because, quite honestly, they're excruciatingly dull. I chose a career on-camera partly so I wouldn't have to sit in meetings. I mean, would you rather interview Will Smith or plan an upcoming commercial shoot for a garage door company? That's what I thought. Yet, there I was, listening to somebody drone on about something I didn't care about and letting my mind wander to negative places.

At one point during the meeting, my producer, Bianca, mouthed the word "stop" to me from across the room. I didn't know why at first until her eyes instructed me to look at my stomach. Turns out, I'd been poking my stomach with one hand while checking my neck lump with the other. I didn't even realize it.

I stopped. A few minutes later, Bianca mouthed "stop" again and aggressively fixed her gaze on my stomach. This time, my shirt was untucked, and my hand moved underneath it, poking my stomach, searching for my liver and any lumps or bumps it might contain. I even did that thing doctors do where they tap your stomach with their fist to locate your liver. I think it is called percussion, and I have no clue if I did it right, but I'm guessing I didn't. I'm not sure if my coworkers saw me because the topic turned to microphone windscreens, so I'm guessing several of them fell asleep. But if they did see me, I can only imagine what they thought. My only hope is that they wrote my behavior off as just "something those weird on-camera people do."

I was rapidly losing my mind, and all this just a few weeks after I felt mentally great. Sadly, my anxiety got worse and my neurosis soon worked its way down to the lower half of my anatomy. I was sitting on my couch one day and had an itch on my left thigh. No big deal just scratch it, which I did, except I noticed that my inner thigh felt swollen. I assumed it was the position I was sitting in, so I moved my leg a bit, but it still felt abnormally big.

Try and guess what my next two moves were. First, I felt my right inner thigh to compare the two (the left one was bigger) and next I searched WebMD to see if the thigh area had lymph nodes. There were indeed a few nodes in the inner thigh/groin region, which instantaneously triggered my next batch of catastrophic thinking. I spent much of that day pressing down on both thighs, even resorting to my favorite fallback of using my fingers as a ruler. As always, I had no idea what I was feeling for, but I could absolutely tell there was an asymmetry and that the muscle (or tissue or fat or lymph nodes or whatever) in my left thigh was bigger than in my right. Here's the thought process that followed:

I'm athletically ambidextrous, and while I throw with my right hand, I kick with my left leg. Is it possible that years of soccer made my left leg stronger? Could be but considering I hadn't played soccer in 20 years—and, by the way, I was a goalie, so I didn't really kick the ball— probably not. Did I get stung by a bee and this was some sort of allergic reaction? I think I would have felt that. Was my left leg always bigger and I just never noticed, because why would a normal, rational human being ever notice something like that? Are some people's legs different sizes? How do they shop for jeans? Was my leg getting bigger because I was touching it? It was certainly getting redder and sorer, but bigger?

I tried to make myself stop touching it but couldn't. In order for me to conduct a proper examination I had to do something about all this leg hair. In 41 years of life I had never shaved my legs. I'd shaved my arms, chest, back, and stomach but never once my legs. That streak came to an ignominious end. Into the shower I went, razor in hand.

Five minutes later I had two super weird patches of smooth skin on my left and right inner thighs. Bizarre to look at; but easier to observe my predicament and formulate a completely unqualified diagnosis.

I couldn't stop dwelling on this, and my legs were tender and raw from the constant poking. So even though I didn't have an oncology appointment scheduled for a month, I made an emergency one and went to see Dr. Lutzky later that week. That bears repeating: I made an emergency oncology appointment to have a doctor look at my thighs. There I sat in the waiting room surrounded by people about to get chemotherapy, and I was there because of tenderized, and possibly asymmetrical thighs.

Dr. Lutzky examined me and did his due diligence before dismissing it as nothing. I'm not sure, but I think he thought I was insane. I thanked him for seeing me, apologized for wasting his time, and limped away searching for the nearest ice packs.

Sadly, the hypochondriasis didn't end there. It had gone from my liver, to my thighs, all the way to my feet; I was going for full-body insanity. One afternoon I sat in a movie theatre (I can't remember the movie, probably because I hardly watched it) rubbing my face and neck to drain the lymphatic fluid, as per my usual. I felt comfortable doing this in a theater, because of the darkness. Plus, people were generally preoccupied with the actual movie, so they never really noticed me. And if they did, they didn't say anything. Plus, if I had to touch myself in a dark movie theater the face and neck seemed like two of the more harmless options.

At one point in the film my foot fell asleep. No big deal, it's happened before. All the other times it happened, like it's probably happened to all of you, it went away on its own. However, it doesn't go away on its own if you obsess about it. And sure enough, if you obsess enough, the other foot might fall asleep too, which is precisely what happened.

I sat in that theater, rubbing my face and neck and kicking both feet against the chair in front of me. This time I'm certain people noticed me. How could they not? I'm surprised security didn't escort me out of there.

When the movie ended, I Googled numb feet, found links to spinal and brain tumors and planned my funeral, for the millionth time. Luckily for me I had my next round of CAT scans coming up, and all these questions would be answered.

CHAPTER 23

The Dolphins Cancer Challenge

In the midst of my total body meltdown, the Miami Dolphins organization held its sixth annual "Dolphins Cancer Challenge," or D.C.C. The organization founded the event in 2010 as its signature initiative, and 100% of the participant-raised funds every year go to innovative cancer research at the Sylvester Comprehensive Cancer Center, where I had my two surgeries.

The Dolphins organization asked me if I would participate in the event, and I eagerly said yes and joined "Team Hurricanes." Not only had I attended the University of Miami for college, but I had a very special place in my heart for the University's Sylvester Comprehensive Cancer Center. I felt honored to be part of that team. And running in a 5K seemed to be the perfect cure for my numb feet.

As a team member, and a cancer survivor, I gave a video

testimonial about my story and the fine care I received at Sylvester. The hospital's public relations staff asked me if I'd be all right if they used my story and picture as part of their promotional campaign. I said sure, assuming they would attribute a quote to me or put my face on a press release or something. Little did I know the picture would be mailed to homes across South Florida and blown up full-sized and plastered all over the walls of the Cancer Center. I became wall art! Anyone who set foot in that hospital got to see a life-size version of me. It was another way for me to give back to the community and spread awareness about my disease, and let people know that late stage melanoma was not a death sentence (even if I needed to be reminded of that from time to time).

I thought the whole experience was super cool, and every now and then friends visiting the hospital took a picture of the mural and sent it to me. I even went back to Sylvester for a routine check-up months later and saw myself, hanging there in the lobby. That was surreal. Way more surreal than seeing myself on TV.

The 2016 "Dolphins Cancer Challenge" raised over five million dollars for cancer research, with a few thousand of that coming from me, my friends, and my family. In total, the event has raised over 16.5 million dollars since its inception in 2010, with all that money going to Sylvester so they can save lives.

The DCC continues to grow and every year I remain part of it, interviewing the event's ambassadors on TV ahead of time and covering it live as I participate in it. Just like the Miles For Melanoma 5K, the DCC brings together a community of cancer warriors. There's solidarity, empathy, love and exercise; it doesn't get much better than that. I hope if you find yourself in a situation similar to mine you attend events like these. I promise you'll be glad you did. And if anyone asks you to share your story, do it. It doesn't matter where you are in your fight, the point is you're fighting. And you have no idea how inspirational that is.

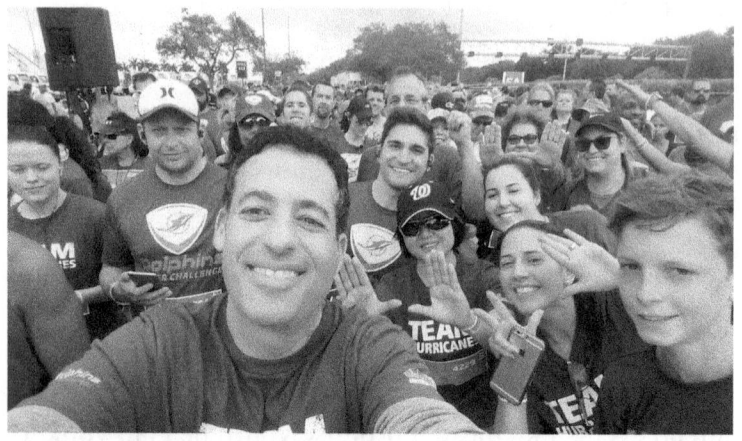

At the Dolphins Cancer Challenge...

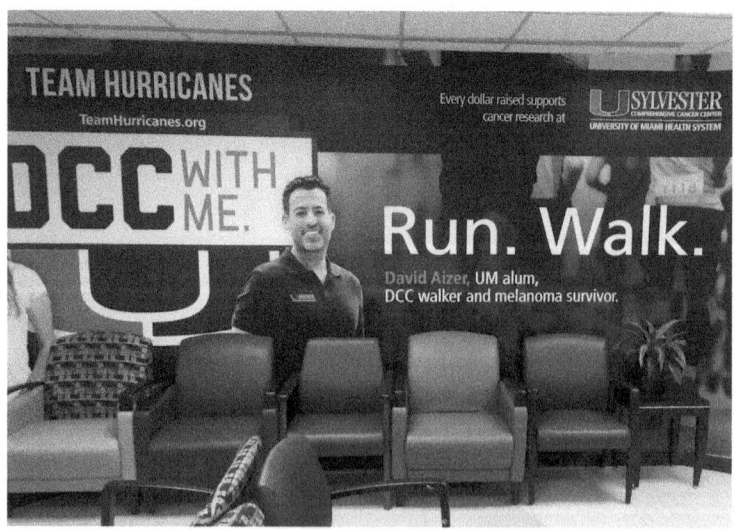

and on the wall at the Sylvester Comprehensive Cancer Center.

CHAPTER 24

The Night Before The Scans

While the DCC was a nice distraction, time, as they say, stops for no one. The calendar turned to April 2016, a year-and-a-half since my initial diagnosis, and I had the next round of scans on my neck, chest, stomach, and pelvis set for the following morning. As usual, that night, I was a disaster. I worried about my neck, my spine, my liver, and, for no reason, my lungs. Although I had made it past each of the individual freak-outs I chronicled in the previous few chapters, they all came roaring back because I knew judgment day was a mere 12 hours away. So that night I wrote down my feelings in a journal.

And I think it would be more powerful if I gave you those words exactly how they poured out of my head that night; rather than try and rewrite them in a different tense. So, here's what I wrote the night before my scans:

"I have scans in 12 hours, and I'm having trouble breathing. Why isn't this getting any easier? I feel no calmer now than I did the night before my scans one year ago, but I totally should. So far, all the scans, oncology appointments, physical exams, and blood tests have been clean. I've been cancer-free for over a year. But instead of that making me feel better, in some ways it's making things worse.

"I can't help but feel that all my good fortune is going to catch up with me. That I've been very lucky so far, but one of these times, maybe tomorrow, my luck will run out and the cancer will return. And I'll get another bad news phone call.

"Thinking this way is so stupid. It suggests that God is out to get me. That he is malicious and wants to bring me short-term joy just so the pain he ultimately brings me will hurt worse. It's such a stupid way to think and it defies logic. If I've been healthy so far, that is a good thing. It means I am more likely to continue to be healthy. It's just common sense. Would I rather have had a relapse already, so I wouldn't have to worry about having one tomorrow?

"I know all this, but I can't stop. I can't turn off my brain. It just seems like every day there's a story about someone who beat cancer only to have it return and kill them. Is tomorrow my turn to hear that news?

"It also doesn't help that earlier today I Googled an

article about the new immunotherapy treatments in the fight against melanoma, and in the article there was the sentence, "Most stage 3 melanoma cases ultimately metastasize to other parts of the body." I'm stage 3. Bad time to read that.

"It's funny because I think back on all the things that used to scare me. Asking a woman out; asking for a raise; getting up to bat in baseball with the game on the line… now those things don't faze me at all. I'm envisioning a scenario where I hit a home run to win the game, ask a woman on a date, and get a big, fat raise from my boss. That day would be way better than this day. But a negative scan result tomorrow would blow that day out of the water.

"It's just the immediacy of it all. You walk into the MRI center totally healthy, at least as far as you can tell. You leave there knowing a radiologist will soon be examining your films, looking for cancer. I'm so lucky that my radiologist is a family friend so I get the results quickly, usually within an hour. I don't envy anyone who has to wait a week or two for these results. That sucks. But that one hour I have to wait will be gut wrenching. Mom and I will go to our usual bagel place after she comes with me to the scans. I'll order my egg-bagel-wrap thing, but I won't be able to eat it. Between the anxiety and the two barium shakes I'll drink when I wake up tomorrow morning, my stomach will be Chernobyl. Those shakes might make it easier to get clear scans, but damn they're horrible. I'd rather drink chalk.

"And of course, I'll be staring at my phone the whole time, waiting for it to ring. Seconds turn to minutes; minutes turn into a half an hour, and still no call. Then it rings, and it's Kenny (my radiologist) and it's the moment of truth. I either do or don't have cancer. That's what I have to look forward to tomorrow.

"Tonight, I'm taking inventory of all the ailments I'm feeling, and I'm imagining the worst: that I've got cancer everywhere, all over my body. I know that a headache can just be a headache and a stomachache can just be a stomachache, but tonight I'm just wondering if it's a brain tumor or a liver tumor or both.

"And the pain in my chest is probably just anxiety. But it could also be a symptom of lung cancer. And I remember one of my doctors telling me a year ago that if my melanoma would metastasize there was a high probability it would go to my lungs. So now I'm afraid I have lung cancer. On top of that, one of my vocal chords hurts and my voice feels weaker than usual. Is it because I went to a concert Saturday night and screamed? Maybe it's throat cancer? Is that better or worse than lung cancer? Better, right? I think I'd rather have that. Doesn't Michael Douglas have that? I think he got it from HPV. Is that what I have?

"I want to call one of my doctor friends and ask for reassurance. I want to know I'm fine right now. But it's late so I can't. What would they say anyway? They won't say I have nothing to worry about and they won't say the cancer is never coming back because they don't know. They'll tell me that's the point of the scans and that I should get some sleep.

"Maybe I'll turn on *Seinfeld*; George Costanza is even worse than me. He'll be good for a laugh.

"You know what—I'm going to be fine tomorrow. This is just pre-exam jitter stuff. I caught it early, it's gone, and it's not coming back. I have great doctors and a great support system, and all the mathematics suggest my cancer isn't coming back. Besides I can't get sick and I can't die. I have too much to do. I need to become the national ambassador in the fight against melanoma. That's why God gave this to me in the first place. So, I'm not going anywhere.

"And if something is wrong with me I'll just beat it anyway. Jimmy Carter is 91, and he had stage 4 melanoma in his brain and liver, and thanks to immunotherapy he's fine. He's building houses and eating peanuts. And I'm in way better shape than that guy is.

"Alright, I got this. I don't even need *Seinfeld*. I'm going to sleep. Tomorrow will be tough but hopefully the next entry I write will be filled with good news and gratefulness. Goodnight, see you tomorrow."

As I re-read what I wrote that night, a few things stand out to me, and hopefully they can help you. The first is to be nice to yourself. I called myself "stupid" multiple times. I wasn't "stupid" for being scared, and you aren't either; even if the doctors tell you "your odds are good." Cancer can come back, that's just a fact. You have every right to be scared.

Also, it's funny how many times I contradicted myself in that passage. That's an indication of how many different emotions you wrestle with as a cancer patient. Everybody processes cancer differently, but those emotions are there in all of us.

Finally, I had begun to accept that this happened to me *on purpose*, that God chose to give me cancer because He (or She) had a plan for me. And my goal is to honor that plan by becoming the national ambassador in the fight against melanoma. Three years later I am working hard to make that a reality. This book is a big part of that plan. Advocacy is a very empowering feeling. I highly recommend it.

CHAPTER 25

The Results Are In

Morning came, and I prepared for the scans. Physically, a CAT scan isn't bad; it's fairly quick and totally painless. I'm on my back, in a long tube, but both ends of the tube are open and my head and feet hang out, alleviating whatever claustrophobic feelings I may have. All the while the imaging machine takes a series of pictures, searching for disease. Halfway through the exam the technician injects me with contrast to highlight certain parts of my body in the images. The contrast gives me an uncomfortably warm sensation as it works its way through my body, but after a few moments the feeling subsides.

Each individual scan takes only a few seconds, and the whole process is over in about 20 minutes. The hardest part is that I'm constantly wondering what the scans are detecting and if the technician sees anything on the computer. When the exam is over, there is a real temptation to ask the techs if they saw anything, and failing that, there's a temptation to try and read their body language, or even their voice. I've asked the tech a few times if they saw anything, and the answer usually is, "I wasn't looking," which I have a feeling isn't true. I would imagine there are many instances when a technician sees cancer and knows right then and there the patient is in trouble. That has to be hard for them.

By comparison, my annual brain MRI is torturous. It is physically, mentally, and emotionally excruciating. First of all, the exam takes about 45 minutes, and I'm on my back the whole time, not allowed to move. Imagine not being able to move for 45 minutes. Even my slightest movement can affect the imaging and, in some cases, render the entire exam moot; which would mean I'd need to come back and do the whole thing all over again. The littlest things, like an itch on your nose, get magnified because you can't do anything about them. Second, my head is enclosed in the tube, so I feel completely trapped and claustrophobic. I know it's not analogous to being buried alive, but that is the sensation it gives me. It feels like there is no escape. Third, the exam is relentlessly loud due to the vibration of the metal coils violently banging away around my head.

My fear of moving, and thereby nullifying the exam, plus the loud, perpetual thumping of the machine surrounding my head, plus the thought that the imaging might be revealing tumors makes the experience brutal. The first time I had a brain MRI I panicked and hyperventilated. I couldn't breathe and wanted to quit so badly, and nearly shouted "stop" a dozen times. It took everything I had, every pep talk I could muster, to get my breath back and stay in that machine until the exam ended. And every single time I finish a brain MRI I'm completely spent, physically, mentally, and emotionally.

A friend once told me to picture myself on the beach to relax during these exams. To me, there are few thoughts less relaxing than the beach with the sun beating down on me, so I try instead to think of all the things I'm grateful for. Gratefulness and prayer get me through my scans.

Back to the morning at hand, and the CAT scans of my neck, chest, abdomen, and pelvis. I somehow got the barium drinks down, while holding my nose to mute the taste, and had my scans. After the exam, my mom and I headed to the usual post-scan bagel place (would you believe I still don't know the name of the restaurant… that's how much of a blur those mornings are) to wait for the results. I ordered my egg-bagel-wrap thing but had no desire to eat it. The barium shakes messed with my stomach, which was already in knots. I didn't want to add anything else to the mix.

My mom, on the other hand, is a nervous eater and she had no trouble scarfing down her bagel sandwich. Even watching her eat made me nauseous. But she finished every bite and moved on to her coffee while I moved on to staring at my cell phone and willing it to ring. That's the thing about cell phones: they never ring when you want them to.

We filled the time by talking. Well, she talked. I sort of listened while fidgeting with my phone settings to make sure I hadn't accidentally set the ringer to silent. At one point I switched it to vibrate, thought better of it, and switched it back to ring. I kept staring at it, and it kept not ringing.

Again, I know how lucky I am that I only have to wait an hour or so for the results of my scans, but that hour, on that day, felt like an eternity.

My mom's also a nervous talker and that morning's agenda included the details of a play she was co-directing, the latest gossip about her mahjong group, and almond milk. Admittedly, I half-listened, with one ear on her and one eye on the phone. I knew she talked to ease her nerves, and to ease mine. I love her for that. And I learned a thing or two about almond milk. She even got bold and asked me about my dating life, but I wasn't having that conversation.

I can't blame her for trying, though.

Then, the phone rang. It was my radiologist, Dr. Stein, with wonderful news.

"David," he said, "everything looks good, my man. No changes." He elaborated on the specifics, and all was as it should be. I had clean scans and once again no cancer. I was good to go!

Elation and relief poured over both me and my mom, and we texted friends and family with the news. No matter how many times you get good news, it never gets old. It's still just as awesome every time. I felt beyond happy to be healthy but also a little silly that I'd obsessed about it the night before, and even mustered a chuckle at my expense. Let's be honest, I was still a hot mess. But, again, if I can't laugh at myself about the throat/lung/liver/stomach cancer episode from the night before the scans, what good is any of this? Hopefully, for all you hypochondriacs out there, you too will be able to enjoy a hearty laugh at your own expense after your own bit of good news. I may have been a wacko, but I was a cancer-free wacko, and I didn't have any more scans for six months. So, any symptoms I felt over those six months would have to wait until the next time I visited the imaging center—or until I measured them myself.

It is amazing how quickly your symptoms go away once you get good news. Once Kenny called me and told me I didn't have cancer, all my aches and pains vanished. My breathing returned to normal and my throat, chest, and stomach stopped hurting. And I decided that the next time my foot went numb in a movie theatre I would just enjoy the damn movie.

I had an eye doctor appointment a few hours after my CAT scans, as part of my clinical trial protocol, and that too turned out to be fine. I was slightly worried because I'd been experiencing some weakness in and around my left eye. It turned out to be nothing and most probably a result of the residual trauma on my facial nerve from the surgeries. Like my sweaty face, it's something I may just have to live with the rest of my life. Annoying, yes, but so what, it's another "battle scar." And if you're ever at a restaurant and see a droopy-eyed guy wiping sweat from his face, come say "hi." I promise I won't bite; that would require too many napkins.

One thing I took from the ophthalmologist appointment, and I want to pass along to you, is how important it is to wear sunglasses. Good sunglasses with UV protection, not the cheap, crappy kind. Melanoma can spread to the eye, but it can also originate there. So, I'll have regular eye exams for the foreseeable future. And this nonsense about me not wearing sunglasses when I play tennis at noon in South Florida because it hinders my game must stop. Can you imagine getting melanoma in your eye because you're worried about your forehand?

"That poor guy has eye cancer. But what a forehand he had. You should have seen it. Of course, he can't see it. He can't see anything."

After the combined good news from my scans and my eye appointment, I found some alone time, prayed and shed a few tears. They were tears of joy, but tears nonetheless. I have embraced my sensitive side through all of this. I used to cry in sad movies. Now I cry in romantic comedies and even some sitcoms. I watched *Love Actually* recently for the millionth time, and it got the tears flowing. Some episodes of *Modern Family* choke me up, too. That darn Phil Dunphy, he has such a huge heart. Why won't his father-in-law love him? Once commercials start making me cry I will officially turn in my man-card.

I'm hoping being emotionally vulnerable makes me charming, or at least offsets my face and eye.

CHAPTER 26

Shots! But Not The Fun Kind

One week after each round of scans I visit the oncology office. I'm using the present tense here because after four years, I'm still getting scans and still seeing the oncologist. We discuss the exam results (even though I already know them), Dr. Lutzky gives me a physical, and the nurses draw my blood. Up until two years ago when my clinical trial ended, the nurses would administer my injections during these visits. So, there I sat in April 2016, a week after the scans, in the waiting room ready to be a lab rat. The good news was, after that visit, I only had four injections left in the trial.

I have this mostly under control by now, but at that time I would get rather anxious sitting in my oncologist's waiting room. Of course, who wouldn't be? It's not exactly Disney World.

It's probably the word "oncologist" that sets people off

in the first place. If he were called "frozen yogurt" I know I'd feel much more relaxed.

I was particularly dreading that visit due to the 12 vials of blood I'd soon be parting with. "Parting with" sounds like I'd be giving them up voluntarily, that was not the case. The nurses would actively take them from me, and I would no doubt feel vial-lated. Different visits required different amounts of blood and this visit would be the biggest outpouring yet. But the physical pain of the needle didn't concern me. I've seen way bigger dudes than me pass out over needles, whereas needles don't send me into a panic. Of course, I think I'm dying if I don't know the words to a song on the radio, so who am I to judge anybody? The part that had me playing mental gymnastics was what the lab technicians might find when they tested my blood. Although I had clean scans, traces of cancer could still be in my body and could show up in the blood work. I had become so conditioned to worrying, it was getting easier and easier to find things to worry about. No cancer in my organs? Awesome. But, maybe it's in my blood. And then it will be in my organs. And then I'll die.

With 12 vials drawn, the techs had a lot of blood to test. This meant that for a few days after my appointment I'd be sitting around waiting for yet another phone call from the hospital, a phone call that may or may not even come, depending on if the news was good or bad. Like I said, there's always something.

The only benefit of my nervousness that day was that I had no trouble providing a urine sample; I probably could have provided two. I overflowed the cup and thought about saving some if I ever needed surgery again. After the urine, I gave blood and went back to the waiting room for my turn to see Dr. Lutzky.

While I waited, I engaged in an internal debate as to whether or not I should ask the doctor a certain question. When I first met Dr. Lutzky in February 2015, he gave me my recurrence rates as well as my five-year and 10-year survival rates. By the way, when you are diagnosed, be prepared to hear those numbers, even if you don't want to. In my experience, with the various oncologists I met, you have to specifically tell them you don't want to know those numbers. Otherwise, they'll tell you. I can see both sides of the argument. On one hand you want to be armed with the data, so you can frame your mindset and expectations accordingly. On the other hand, those numbers are in fact, just numbers. They aren't you. They include "all comers," meaning people who may have had a myriad of other health problems in addition to cancer. Their outcome doesn't preordain your outcome. So, again, I can understand why somebody would want to know, or not know, their survival rates.

At the time of my diagnosis, according to the numbers, the chance of my melanoma recurring was somewhere around 30%, my five-year survival rate was roughly 70% and my ten-year survival rate was around 55%, slightly better than a coin flip. While these were apparently good numbers for stage 3 melanoma, they still scared the hell out of me. I mean, previous to getting cancer, the chance of melanoma recurring was 0% and I'm guessing my five-year general survival rate was probably around 95%.

As I waited to see him, I kicked around if I should ask him if my recurrence rate and survival rate had changed. It had been a year since my clinical trial started so one part of me figured those numbers had gotten better. On the other hand, melanoma most often recurs within the first two to three years, and as it was early on in year two, perhaps I had just entered the danger zone. I knew one thing for sure: if I did ask, his answer would either make or ruin my day. To continue the frozen yogurt metaphor, it would either be cookies and cream or tart. Sorry if you like tart yogurt, I just don't get it.

As I sat there debating I looked around the waiting room and realized that cancer doesn't discriminate. I was the youngest patient there—which I usually am—and that used to send me into a bit of a pity party. But I'd gotten past that; after all, there are kids with cancer. They have it much worse than me.

The room housed black people, white people, elderly people, and Latin-American people. There were melanoma patients, breast cancer patients, lung cancer patients, and more. Cancer extends its hellacious reach to everyone. It can touch us all, and we're all in this together.

Ultimately, a nurse summoned me and led me to the exam room: one step closer to Dr. Lutzky. Most people get frustrated by how long it takes to see the doctor. From start to finish, I usually spend about two to three hours at the oncologist's office. If I'm being honest I don't mind the long doctor visits, because they keep me out of the office. I'm not saying I'm glad I got cancer, so I could skip out on my job; I'm just saying it's a tiny little ancillary benefit. I know television host sounds like a super cool job. And mostly it is. But my job isn't all about interviewing South Florida celebrities and sipping champagne on yachts with South Beach models. Although, that would be nice. Instead there's quite a bit of minutiae and office work and who wants to deal with that when you're trying to enjoy the preciousness of every day. That said, if I'm choosing a cancer exam, blood work, and painful injections over an afternoon at my job it might be time to look for a new place to work.

After a while Dr. Lutzky came in, we exchanged pleasantries, he sat down at his computer and accessed my electronic file. Every time he does that he reads it in silence, which is obviously totally normal, but I must admit the silence gets to me. I can't help but try and read his facial expressions. I know what he's looking at – the results of the scans – but maybe he's studying something else? Something I don't already know? Maybe there's something in the report that concerns him?

He sat there in silence, looking at the computer, and then asked, "Wait a minute, what is this, here?"

I almost jumped off the exam table when I heard that. His question even got the attention of the very sweet clinical trial administrator, Diane Chambers (she has the same name as the character from *Cheers*, which I took as a good sign because that was my favorite childhood show).

"What?" Diane said.

Dr. Lutzky replied, "Why can't I advance the screen?"

Dude! Come on! I thought I was dying! I flashed back to when the American Red Cross called me and asked how me to spell my last name.

After tech support intervened, we made it past that horrific moment and the rest of the exam went smoothly—save for some weird small talk on my part. In doctors' offices I'm a nervous talker and always feel the need to chat with my physicians about their social lives, kids, and hobbies. I do care about the answers; my doctors have become my extended family.

I asked him about my diet, my social drinking regimen, and even about the ingredients in sunscreen. Essentially, I was eating fine, drinking in appropriate moderation, and the benefits of sunscreen far outweighed any of its risks. I asked him about all the vials of blood I gave, and he explained they could indicate abnormal levels in my liver and kidneys and some other medical stuff I really didn't understand. It would be at least two days until he had those results, which meant two days of high anxiety for me, pondering all potential outcomes and staring at my phone again, wondering if it would ring.

And then Dr. Lutzky gave me great news. I asked him about survival rates and recurrence percentages, but I told him I didn't want to know any numbers, only if I should feel any more confident than I did a year ago. He reiterated what I had previously read, which is that the highest recurrence rate occurs in the first three years. But what he told me, that I *didn't already know*, and what put me in a great mood the rest of the day, was that my three-year clock actually started from my initial diagnosis in January, 2015, *not* in April of that year, when my clinical trial began.

Instead of being one year into survivorship, I was actually one year and three months into it. I know it's only a 90-day difference, but it felt amazing.

After the exam I headed to the treatment room for the last stop on my oncology tour: the clinical trial shots—one in each arm and one in each leg. I always hated that part of the process the most. Not because of the shots, but because there I would see other patients undergoing various forms of chemotherapy. Some looked sicker than others; in fact, some looked terribly sick. Luckily my mom, my rock in all this, sat by my side that day as she did, and still does, for every scan and every oncology appointment.

While I am grateful for her support, I don't know why she kept putting herself through my injections; the shots seemed to hurt her more than they hurt me, and she didn't even get them. But I'm her baby, her now 44-year-old baby, and my pain is her pain. And if I tell her not to come to an appointment it will devastate her. We're a package deal at this point.

I used to worry, for no good reason, that I might accidentally get a different patient's shots, despite the numerous protocols to prevent that from happening. They ask for your name and birthday three times. I mean, I appreciate the attention to detail but I'm clearly not the 90-year-old woman sitting next to me. My name is not Edna. Even for my level of neurosis, me accidentally getting the wrong medicine seemed ridiculous, so I stopped concerning myself with that. Ironically, the thing I should have concerned myself with was the possibility I could be getting a placebo, but since I made up my mind in the beginning that my trial had the active drug I never gave it a second thought.

Truth be told, the shots did hurt quite a bit. That's because they were intradermal: meaning injected into the dermis, just below the surface of my skin, and that area has a lot of nerves. A deeper injection would have hurt less. But I couldn't complain about the pain that day because sitting next to me, separated only by a curtain, a lady sobbed as she received her chemo. And that broke my heart.

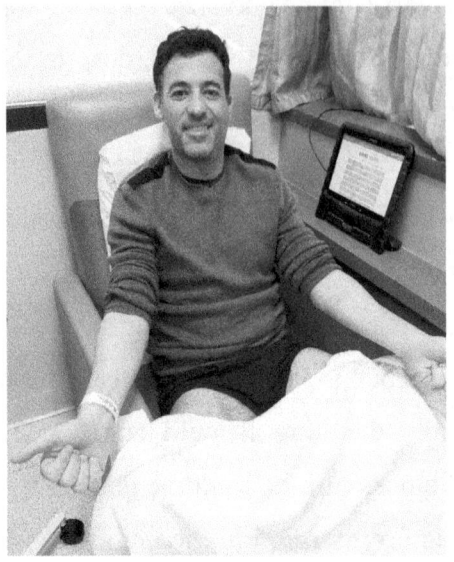

Getting my injections: one in each arm and one in each leg.

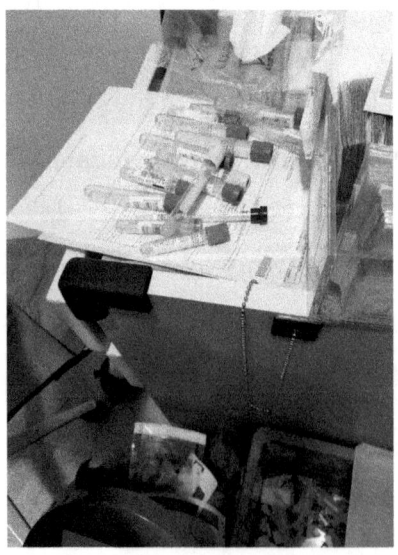

All those vials are about to be full.

CHAPTER 27

Shopping At The (Anion) Gap

Typically if the bloodwork is normal I don't hear from Dr. Lutzky or anyone in the oncology department. I get an email after a few days notifying me that my results are available electronically, but I don't look at them. Mostly because, and this may shock you, I'm not a doctor. However, I did have some anxiety four days after this appointment because I had asked Diane to email me when the results were in, even if they were good, just so I could get closure. I did that from time to time, typically when there was a lot of blood drawn, and she was always great about it. But on this occasion I hadn't heard from her for four days. Granted, it was now Sunday and two of those days were the weekend and that shouldn't count, but that made far too much sense for me. Plus, since my cancer diagnosis I had gotten a fair amount of medical news on weekends, so a precedent did exist.

Of course, I hadn't heard from Dr. Lutzky either and

I figured he'd be the one to tell me bad news, so I took that as a good sign. The results probably hadn't come in yet. Or, perhaps, they had come in, I was fine, and there was no reason for a phone call. Or, maybe I was dying, and the oncology center didn't want to ruin my weekend. Maybe they were saving the really bad news for Monday morning. Mondays suck anyway; why not just tell me then? I needed to know!

I had emailed Diane at 9 p.m. on Friday night asking for an update, which admittedly is rude and not fair to her. When she didn't reply (probably because she has a life) that caused me even more distress. So, I was regretting every part of that decision.

On Sunday night, I received an email. It wasn't from Diane; it was from Mount Sinai Medical Center, letting me know the results were in fact in, and I could review them electronically. As mentioned, I had never reviewed my chart before because I didn't know what the numbers meant and, knowing me, I'd figure out a reason to freak out about one of them. But screw it, I decided to look. I accessed my electronic file and clicked on "my results."

It's a dicey proposition to give a hypochondriac access to his own medical files and lab results before he talks to his doctor about them. My initial thought was that Dr. Lutzky must have seen the results on Friday and signed off on them, thereby releasing them electronically. I mean, there's no way the oncology department would send me results if they hadn't been cleared first, right? Could they do that?

I thought it over and changed my mind, and decided not to look. It was Sunday night, I could wait until the morning. Surely I would hear from somebody then. Or maybe I'd just die in my sleep and wouldn't have to deal with it. I felt at peace with that decision…for 15 seconds…then picked up my phone, opened the page, and accessed my results. Time to play doctor, just not in the high school way.

I saw a bunch of words with numbers next to them that represented different levels of different things inside my body. Pretty good analysis, right? And that's without medical school.

As I started down the list, I developed a system, almost right away. I didn't even look at the words; I just looked at the number next to each word to see if it landed in the specified range.

To my joy, every number landed in the range. Well, almost every number. Towards the end of the third page I found one number below the normal range. Damn it! I was doing so well. I almost made it. The number belonged to something called the Anion Gap, and mine was a 9.1, with the minimum number in the range being 10.

Oh, no. Not the dreaded Anion Gap. And mine is low. That's it, I'm done for. Nobody survives a low Anion Gap.

Wait a second, what the hell was an Anion Gap? It sounded like a place in Colorado where people ski, not something inside my body. So, naturally, I had to Google Anion Gap. Turned out it had something to do with electrolytes. I didn't read much more out of fear I would read something I didn't like. Like, "A low Anion Gap means certain death, especially in melanoma patients. Often, the patient spontaneously explodes." Something like that.

Then I started to wonder if my clinical trial had affected my Anion Gap or maybe I had been born with a low Anion Gap. I could have accessed previous lab results to check those numbers for consistency, but I thought I might stumble upon something else and that would open three or four new cans of worms I wanted no part of, so I chose not to do that.

Then I remembered that Gatorade has electrolytes, and if mine were low perhaps I was dehydrated? That's what Michael Jordan used to tell me in those commercials. And if I was dehydrated then maybe my kidneys weren't working the right way. And if my kidneys weren't working, then…you get where this is going. I went from deciding not to check the results, to checking them, to finding a whole bunch of good results, to finding one that was slightly low, to kidney cancer. This all transpired in five minutes.

And then, I changed my mind again. Screw it, I was already in my medical records, I might as well look at my results from three months ago; cans of worms be damned. I opened my previous results, went right to the Anion Gap and sure enough I had a low number then too. It was 9.6 to be exact. The number was low then and even lower now. I did not like the way the arrow was trending on my Anion Gap. Next time around I might be in the 8's.

I worried about it some more and debated doing additional research. I paced around my apartment, stared into the mirror for a "you're better than this" pep talk and even did some pushups. And then, just as I decided to do more research, a new episode of *Game of Thrones* started and that was arguably even more important than my Anion Gap. So, I left it alone, and figured I'd deal with it the next day.

The moral of the story: if you find yourself about to do extended medical research, opt for Jon Snow instead. He'll save you. I realize roughly four of you reading this may not know who Jon Snow is. You need to fix that. It's *Game of Thrones*, people!

Sure enough I heard from Diane bright and early on Monday. I was indeed "all good." No cancer and, as far as I knew, no concerns over my low Anion Gap. This meant I could officially close the book on that round of scans, exams, and blood work and leave cancer alone for a few months. Another bullet dodged. Incidentally, I never brought up, or thought about, my Anion Gap again and I have no idea how my levels are now.

As I write chapter after chapter about falling apart I'm scared that I'm scaring you, the reader. My purpose for writing this book is to give anyone in this situation some comfort; that even if you have just received terrible news, cancer or otherwise, humor can be your friend. You can make it through your days, even the worst of them. It will be hard, and some days it may feel impossible, but you can do it. Just take it one day at a time, and try to do one positive thing every day.

I feel like I'm doing just the opposite, and I am not reassuring you at all. But I want you to know I AM better today than I was yesterday. And I am way better right now in 2019 than when I got those blood results in 2016. And I will be better tomorrow than I am today. I am absolutely 100% on the road to recovery, and I'm about to get into all of that. And if I can get better, you certainly can as well.

I will tell you though, and this is very important, take care of your mental and physical health from day one. Learn to meditate, go to therapy, exercise, laugh, and love. Figure out what works for you. Do these things even when you don't want to do any of them; in fact, do them *especially* when you don't want to do any of them. Because your body can only handle so much anxiety before it rebels against you. And you and your body need to be on the same team.

For all my anxiety, I am physically stronger and fitter than I have ever been. As I mentioned, every time I feel scared about the cancer coming back I do push-ups. It's my way of knocking the cancer out of me. And although I don't eat great, I do eat better than I used to, most of the time anyway. Do what you can. Understand there will be tough days and ride them out. Just be gentle with yourself.

And whatever you do, keep those electrolytes up. Your Anion Gap is really important…I think.

CHAPTER 28

I'm Flattered, But I Won't Touch Your Mole

As had become my custom, I jumped back into advocacy to rediscover my mojo. But this time, the experience would have an even more profound effect on me and the results of it would be permanent. Shortly after my Anion Gap ordeal, the American Cancer Society of Broward County was set to hold its annual fundraising gala. I very badly wanted to be part of it, so I reached out to the ACS's marketing department and asked if I could attend. I shared my story over the phone, and the department heads invited me to their headquarters to chat. This kicked off an incredible relationship with the American Cancer Society, one I hold very dear to this day. We decided we would work together in multiple capacities going forward. In the following months, I interviewed members of the ACS on television multiple times, and spoke at some of their events, including the gala.

Speaking to the group of melanoma survivors at the "Miles for Melanoma" 5K ignited something in me. I knew I had to do more of that. It was my mission. And this gala would have some very powerful and very wealthy people in the room; people who could open their hearts and checkbooks to donate money to beat cancer. How much money they would donate would be determined, in some small part, by my ability to tug on their heartstrings during my speech.

Forget the donors; the most intimidating people at the gala would be the doctors and oncologists. Sure, they'd be sympathetic toward my plight. They hated cancer too; that's why they would attend. But when you speak in front of them you'd better have your facts straight. The night of the gala, before I spoke, I went over my speech again and again. I had it down stone cold. I was going to own that room.

However, right before I went on stage, a woman who had beaten cancer FIVE times shared her story. There wasn't a dry eye in the house. How on earth could I follow that? It's like watching The Beatles, and then sticking around to see Milli Vanilli. Okay, maybe not Milli Vanilli, maybe Michael Bolton. But definitely not The Beatles. By the way, youngsters, Google Milli Vanilli. You'll be glad you did. And if you're reading this book in 20 years, do whatever has replaced Google.

Can you imagine that: beating cancer five times! It wasn't even one cancer that kept coming back; she had five different types of cancer. And, according to what doctors have told her, because of her DNA she is susceptible to getting cancer again and again. She may have to battle different forms of the disease throughout her life.

What an amazing story, for sure, and she lived to share it. The compassionate, empathetic person in me felt so happy for her and so moved by her words. The performer in me felt bummed I had to speak next. What could I possibly say to move the needle?

I could only imagine the audience's reaction to my story.

"Yeah, yeah, cancer one time, a couple of surgeries, you freak out a lot, and you sweat when you eat. When's dessert?"

Could you get booed off an American Cancer Society stage for having a lame story? I surely hoped not.

So, I downed a vodka soda, kissed my date, and up I went. A quick note: my date that night was a doctor. I had dated a few doctors and nurses since my diagnosis. It made sense because it combined my love of powerful women with my love of asking medical questions about me. However, it never seemed to work out, probably because a woman can only check her date's liver so many times before it becomes annoying.

When I reached the stage the first thing I did was congratulate the lady who spoke before me. She truly is remarkable, and we have become friends. Then I chronicled what I had been through from diagnosis to that very moment. I spoke from the heart, and I learned that having cancer isn't a competition; it doesn't matter how many times you've had it or where it is or what stage it is. Cancer is cancer. It sucks. And it touches everybody, directly or indirectly. The love I felt in that room I will never, ever forget.

After my speech there were tears in the house, not as many as she got, but I saw some tissues. I got a nice ovation and was greeted with incredible warmth. I met a lot of great people that night, and what I found most impactful was that many of them thanked me for reminding them to visit their dermatologist.

Then, as is a continuing theme in this book, things got weird. One of the guys in the audience was drunk; more like wasted, so let's give him the benefit of the doubt for what came next. He approached me a few minutes after my speech, extended his hand, and congratulated me on beating cancer. He then turned the handshake into a hug. He then kissed my cheek. Things were moving at a very uncomfortable pace. I looked to my date for help but she was too busy laughing, as were a few of her friends.

Next, the man asked me about my mole and what it looked like and at what point I decided to go to the doctor. I gave him my answers, and sincerely wished him well, but that didn't end the conversation. Instead, he said, "I see" and took off his tuxedo jacket and started unbuttoning his shirt, right in the middle of the banquet hall. Before I could file a restraining order, or throw dollar bills at him, he asked me to check the mole on his back to see if it was cancerous. In a room full of oncologists this guy asked *me* for my medical opinion.

I explained to him that I was not a doctor, and he should probably put his clothes back on and get the mole checked. In fact, I suggested he make an appointment with any of the 30 physicians at the bar. Disappointed in my diagnosis, he went off in a huff. I never got paid for that consultation.

That actually happens to me quite a bit. Typically, when I tell someone my melanoma story two things occur: first, they express genuine concern and then, and I can actually see this happen on their faces, they zone out (sometimes while I'm mid-sentence) and start thinking about their own moles and if they should see their doctor. I don't mind when this happens, because I want everyone to go to the dermatologist; it's just entertaining to watch the moment they stop listening to me.

Invariably, they'll circle back around to ask me questions about my mole: partly because they're curious and partly to compare it to theirs. And then they'll ask me to look at their mole, sometimes even touch it, to see if it's cancerous. I tell them the same thing every time: go to the doctor.

And yes, I realize the irony, considering how much time I've spent asking friends and family to look at, and touch, various parts of my body. But at least in my case, I always end up going to a professional.

In case you do want to do a self-exam, problematic moles typically follow the ABCDE system: asymmetry, border irregularity, color that isn't uniform, diameter greater than 6 millimeters, and evolving shape, size or color. While this is a good rule of thumb, my melanoma was less than one millimeter. So, the best advice is to go to the dermatologist annually and let a professional figure it out. And stop asking me to touch your mole.

CHAPTER 29

My Shot At Major League Glory

About a month after the American Cancer Society event another local organization opened its doors and heart to me: the Miami Marlins Major League Baseball team. In June 2016, I got to throw out the first pitch at a Marlins' game against the Pittsburgh Pirates as a guest of honor on "Melanoma Awareness Night."

In South Florida you can never educate people too much about taking the proper sun precautions, as this is one of the most at-risk places in the world for skin cancer. But even armed with that knowledge a lot of South Floridians brush off the message and seek out that perfect tan, although it could end up killing them. In fact, instead of sunscreen, South Floridians often wear tanning oil. There's a lot of pressure to look great down here, as ridiculous as that sounds. Also, there's a misconception that melanoma doesn't happen to young people. That it's an "old person's disease" so why should young people have to worry about it? I felt that way before I was diagnosed. But it's not the case. In fact, melanoma is the leading cause of cancer death in women ages 25-30.

It was a big night at the ballpark as the Marlins recognized a handful of melanoma survivors, including myself, during an on-field ceremony before the game. They even held a 50/50 raffle where fans bought tickets for baseball-related items and half the money went to the Melanoma Research Foundation. A huge amount of credit for the entire evening goes not only to the Marlins but to an 18-year-old named Rachel Thomas.

A few years ago, Rachel lost her cousin to melanoma. Since that day, from when she was barely a teenager, Rachel has made it her mission to raise money to cure the disease. I am quite sure we will all hear amazing things from that young lady in the years to come. Rachel brought the idea of a melanoma awareness evening to the Marlins. To see a teenager so passionate about something like that, to the point where she can get a Major League Baseball team to devote a night to it, is a beautiful sight to behold.

So, it all came together, and the Marlins asked me to throw out the first pitch. I said yes not only to support the cause but also to achieve a measure of redemption. I had thrown out the first pitch for the Marlins twice before (a perk of being on television) and neither time went well.

As a guy who pitched all through little league I can honestly say my first two ceremonial first pitches stunk. The first time I threw the ball from the grass in front of the mound (where a senior citizen might throw it), and the second time I threw it from the mound, but in front of the pitching rubber, and it barely eked its way across home plate. I like to think of myself as an athlete, so this was grossly unacceptable.

Upon hearing the news I'd again be throwing out the first pitch, I practiced, a lot. Since I didn't have a catcher on demand, I threw a bunch of baseballs against a tennis court fence. I threw so many balls I hurt my shoulder. But I felt determined to not just throw a good first pitch; I had to throw a great first pitch. I would bring the heat. Of course, heat is a relative term. Compared to how fast major leaguers throw, my "heat" would feel more like room temperature.

By the way, if you ever do throw out a first pitch, it's important to realize that the only person who cares about it is you. It's not like the Marlins had a scout sitting behind home plate. Nobody was offering me a contract when it was over. You throw it, the crowd claps, you shake the catcher's hand, and you leave the field. That's the whole thing, right there. Unless of course you throw it very badly; in which case you wind up on YouTube, but I really hoped that wouldn't happen.

People say it's easy to throw a first pitch, but what they don't realize is that there are thousands of fans watching you, and you get no warm-ups to loosen your arm. You go out there cold, and you only get one shot at it. (I know, I know…it sounds like I'm making excuses. Leave me alone, I'm fragile). Anyway, on gameday I was ready. Nothing would stand in the way of an awesome first pitch. Until they brought out my catcher, and it was Billy The Marlin.

The freaking mascot! Billy The Freaking Marlin! Not the team's starting catcher, or backup catcher, or bullpen catcher, or even the 4th string left fielder; nope, a guy in a ridiculous fish costume and enormously oversized glove would catch my first pitch. He could barely squat in that outfit and definitely did not have a regulation mitt. How could he possibly handle my fastball?

There I stood, on the mound, ready to throw, but distracted by thoughts of the mascot and his ability, or lack thereof, to catch. But like any great pitcher in game seven of the World Series (that's how seriously I took this)

I blocked out the distractions, took a deep breath, and threw that ball as hard as I could.

It landed right over the plate, a perfect strike, my moment of glory…and Billy The Marlin dropped it. A fastball at the knees, and it squirted away from his comically huge glove. My poor first pitch rolled towards the backstop harmlessly.

Yes, I know, it was an honor just to throw out the first pitch. We raised a lot of money for the Melanoma Research Foundation and gave away thousands of bottles of sunscreen to fans in attendance. And in the grand scheme of things my first pitch was *so* not a big deal. But come on, man, you've got to catch that. You're better than that, Billy The Marlin.

Still though, it proved to be an awesome night. One more wonderful thing to come from that experience was that I made a new friend at the game: T.J. Sharpe. T.J. is a stage 4 melanoma survivor and he's become not only a buddy but a source of strength and inspiration for me. In the year 2000, T.J. had a melanoma removed from his collarbone and some lymph nodes from under his arm. The doctors told him they caught it early, and he would be fine, so he went about his life. Twelve years after that, he went to the ER with a spiking fever. Turned out, the melanoma had spread to his lungs, his liver, spleen, and abdomen.

His oncologist told T.J. he' be surprised if he survived two years. Well, seven years later, after multiple surgeries and clinical trials, T.J.'s cancer is essentially gone, and he is completely healthy.

T.J. is now a workout warrior: he bikes, he lifts weights, and he practices yoga. He's even a competitive triathlete. He's also created his own blog called "Patient #1" about his journey with the disease. He and I have a motivational speaking platform together, sharing our stories with advocacy groups, students, doctors, clinical trial administrators and anybody who will listen.

What T.J. has been through has given me a tremendous amount of perspective. When I feel down or scared, I think about T.J.'s courage and it picks me up and empowers me to fight. He probably doesn't know how much he's impacted me, until now. So, thanks, T.J.

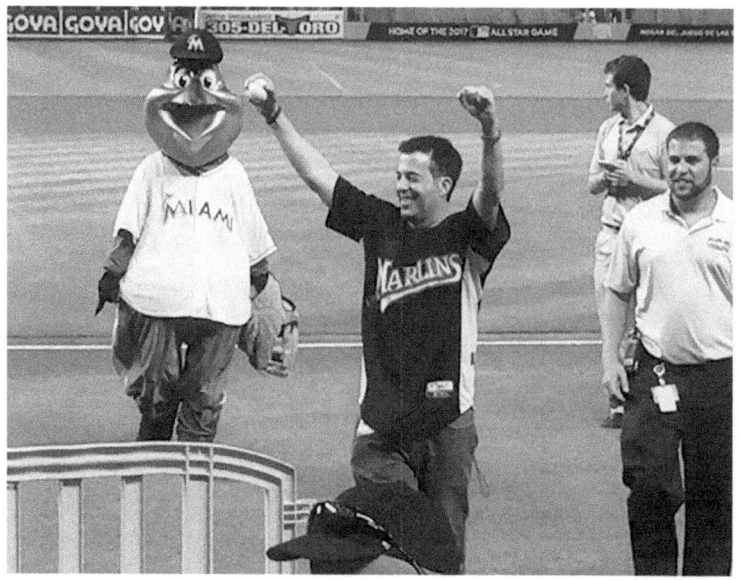

It was a strike! Who could catch with that glove?

CHAPTER 30

Redemption Vacation

Feeling energized and optimistic, I decided to take another crack at a vacation. The Punta Cana experience left a bad taste in my mouth (which I suppose could have been mouth cancer) and I wanted a do-over. So, since one tropical vacation clearly wasn't enough for a melanoma survivor, I doubled down and headed to Club Med Turks and Caicos in August. And let me tell you, it was awesome.

Sure it was hot and sunny, but I wore sunscreen and a hat. I laid out on the beach, daring the sun to mess with me. I played tennis in the middle of the day, wearing sun protective clothing. I drank great wine and ate whatever I wanted. I met people from all over the world and listened way more than I talked, and I learned so much about their cultures.

When I arrived at the hotel I unpacked, and metaphorically put all my troubles into the empty suitcase. I closed the suitcase, stashed it in the closet, and made a deal with myself not to think about that suitcase for a week. Same thing with my cellphone. I put it in the safe on day one and detached from my life in South Florida. It was a wonderfully liberating feeling to be "normal" again, even for just a few days. But it wasn't "normal" as in life before cancer. It was my new normal, after cancer, which was moving increasingly towards advocacy and inspiration and away from anxiety and depression. I soaked in every second of joy on that trip and was so appreciative of my good fortune to be there.

That's not to say I didn't have fleeting moments of hypochondriasis. It was exceedingly hot, so I drank a lot of water, which meant several trips to the men's room. And the constant urination made me wonder if I had prostate cancer, which led me to imagine urology visits and prostate exams, which certainly didn't excite me, but those moments of insanity passed and were replaced by margaritas. Not that I'm advocating drinking to ignore your symptoms, I'm just saying when on an island vacation, chill out and grab a cocktail.

Another reason that vacation meant so much to me is that it's where I started this book. I had been journaling since diagnosis and was writing down notes whenever I could, but I never set my mind to organizing those thoughts. But there, in paradise, so grateful to be alive, I figured this was the perfect place to start.

The only thing missing from that vacation was somebody wonderful to share it with. That was on my to do list for when I got home, as was something else. Something I had neglected for far too long. It was time to go back to therapy.

CHAPTER 31

The Benefits Of Therapy

Upon returning from vacation, I was truly motivated, once and for all, to commit to changing my behavior. Sure, I was heading in the right direction thanks to advocacy, but I still had far too many moments of panic. I couldn't truly "live" if I was going to live like this. It was time to commit to fixing it. Besides, I was running out of body parts to obsess about. I dug in deep and went back to see my therapist, Dr. Ellis, and with his help I finally made real progress.

Before Dr. Ellis did anything else he reassured me it was okay for me to feel like I was spinning out of control. It didn't make me weak that I couldn't mentally "beat this thing." I had gone through the most terrifying experience of my life, by far, and I wasn't inferior or less-than for not being "over it." I deserved credit for choosing advocacy and inspiring others. I needed to remind myself of that and be kinder to myself in the process.

We explored my relationship with God and the comfort I could draw from that. Dr. Ellis reminded me that this was too much to bear on my own, and even though my family and friends were great, there were some things not even they could help me overcome. I learned to lean on God to watch out for me and take over for me when things got too tough. To this day, I thank God all the time for the blessings I've received and for my ability to help others, and I know God will have a hand in whatever I accomplish the rest of my life. If you don't believe in God, try to find someone, or something, to rely on for faith and guidance. You can't do this alone, we all need help.

Another thing I really needed to work on was to change the way I framed my thoughts about the disease. Instead of me giving cancer all the power, I wanted to have power over it. And if I couldn't accomplish that, I at least wanted to make peace with it.

Sure, I had been doing public speaking and non-profit work and I loved that, but I needed to do even more. For that to happen, I needed to believe with 100% conviction that the reason I got melanoma, and survived it, was no accident. I needed to believe that it happened *specifically to me*, so I could be an engine in the fight against the disease. It was my purpose.

Dr. Ellis taught me to frame the conversation differently when I spoke about melanoma. Instead of a problem, it became a challenge. Instead of a disease, I worked on calling it an opportunity. I now had an opportunity to use my platform as a television host, writer, and public speaker to educate as many people as I could and to save as many lives as I could. Stage 3 melanoma wouldn't kill me; it would make me stronger, more present, and more grateful.

And if it came back I would beat it. And if it came back and I couldn't beat it, then I would die. There would be nothing I could do about it. We all die. Not to sound morbid, but for all I know I could also get hit by a truck or struck by lightning. But for as long as I lived I would need to do everything I could to make every second of every day count.

Dr. Ellis also helped me realize so many other things, like how lucky I was that I had something that could in fact be beaten. Some people die suddenly, without any warning, without any doctors on hand. But in my case, I saw a mole, caught before it spread massively, and had great medical care. The fact that it started on my face wasn't a bad thing at all; it was actually a very good thing.

Make no mistake, my face has scars and some asymmetry and my eye still sags. It will never look exactly as it did, especially to me. I've had to overcompensate for it on camera, and I'm self-conscious about it. But, because the mole was on my face it was easier for me to find, thus making me more proactive about getting it removed. Had it been on the back of my leg I might not have seen it or cared about it until it was too late.

And not that it's ever a good time to get cancer, but late-stage cancer isn't a death sentence anymore. A few years ago, a stage 4 melanoma diagnosis meant death, as did many stage 3 diagnoses. Now, more and more people are living with, and beating, this disease as well as breast cancer, lung cancer, and more. There are so many great drugs out there and cures may be on the way in the next few years. So, the trick is to just stay alive for as long as you can because the medicine keeps getting better.

All in all, Dr. Ellis helped me realize that I had a tough circumstance, but it could have been much worse. I had a lot for which to be thankful, and a lot of life left to live. His words allowed me to stop feeling like a victim, and I worked hard to implement that philosophy.

Of course, to this day I still have tough moments, and I'm scared from time to time. I don't want to make it sound like it was that easy to change my perspective. I am continuing to evolve, and I imagine I will do so for the rest of my life. But at least now when I have those tough moments and I'm scared of a relapse, I fall back on what I learned in therapy and I remind myself of my purpose.

But as Dr. Ellis's words started to sink in, I experienced one final test.

CHAPTER 32

Holy Moley: A New Mole!

In December 2016 I had just turned 42. I was approaching two years since my initial diagnosis, and with every day I was feeling better, both mentally and physically. I was at my strongest point since this all started. I'd had another round of clean scans and blood work, had no symptoms, real or otherwise, and I had even stopped checking the lymph nodes under my armpits every morning in the shower.

I was actively applying the lessons Dr. Ellis taught me and feeling rejuvenated. I enjoyed work more. I spent more time with friends. I exercised every day. The only time I mentioned melanoma out loud was as an inspirational tool.

And then, I took my shirt off in front of the mirror.

Standing there shirtless, I noticed a suspicious looking mole on my back. The mole appeared to be new. Not only that, but it looked black. And that's often a bad color for moles.

Okay, let's not panic. I'm sure it's nothing. People get new moles all the time. At least it's not multi-colored.

But a closer look revealed both black and brown coloring.

Damn it, black and brown! That's not good. Alright, relax, you're fine. At least it's flat.

But I ran my finger over it and it felt raised.

Damn it! It's raised and multicolored! This is REALLY not good. Okay, don't freak out. Remember what you've learned. Relax. You're fine, just...don't...freak...out.

Too late, I was freaking out.

My mind raced a thousand miles per hour. I wondered if my dermatologist had seen it during my last visit. Either he hadn't seen it, and it was new, which scared me, or he had seen it, but it had since grown, which also scared me. I seemed screwed in either scenario.

How could I have another one of these things? I had hardly been in the sun the past two years. I looked like an albino vampire. The ever-destructive game of "why me" raged anew in my head. I thought, "Why a new mole and why now?"

Um, God, where are you? Why aren't you answering my phone calls? I thought we had a deal!

I had finally gotten my mojo back, and now I was getting blasted with what could be another melanoma. Granted, this could all be nothing, but I didn't know if I could handle another cancerous mole. At that point a new melanoma would have been harder to deal with than if I'd had a recurrence from my original one. I had mentally prepared myself for that; this I hadn't even considered.

Besides, how many people beat melanoma once, let alone twice?

The rest of the night I alternated between anxiety and anger. I found myself reverting to a lot of the behaviors I thought I had abandoned: staring at the mole over and over, checking WebMD for an amateur diagnosis, and looking at pictures of melanomas to compare them with mine. That's a very ugly Google search by the way. If you ever want to scare your kids, that's a good way to do it.

I really tried to be calm, reciting aloud some of the mantras Dr. Ellis gave me, but it was an uphill battle. I wrote those mantras down and said them over and over, to get them to resonate. I was trying everything I could think of to stay poised. I even reverted to middle of the night pushups.

I woke up in the morning, shook off the cobwebs, gave myself a pep talk and resolved to be an optimist. I was going to be fine. It was just a mole, and this was just a character builder. I called the dermatologist's office, booked an appointment for that afternoon and set out for the day.

When I got to work I figured that because of my

color-blindness perhaps I misjudged the mole and it wasn't multicolored at all. I mean, the mole resided on my back, so I didn't have the best angle to see it anyway. I needed another opinion—in addition to the one I'd soon get from a licensed medical doctor. So, I lifted my shirt and asked Bianca to check it out. Granted, this is precisely what the stranger did to me at the American Cancer Society benefit and I just made fun of him for that. But, whatever, it's my book not his.

You might think lifting my shirt at work and asking a woman to check my bare back would be a human resources violation. And in many places, it might be. But in a television studio we're all a little weird. You have to be a little off to work in TV. It's a bizarre industry. Bianca had helped apply makeup to my sty and she had felt the cyst on my forehead. She was part of my medical team.

Bianca confirmed the mole did indeed look black-ish-brown and elevated; the dreaded double-whammy. I officially had zero chance of being productive at work that morning, unless you count looking at pictures of black-brown moles productive.

Two p.m. finally arrived, and I saw Dr. Bernhardt. When I showed him my back all I wanted to hear was, "You're fine. It's nothing. It's the most boring thing I've seen all day."

That, by the way, is one of my favorite expressions of his. He says that from time to time when I show him something that concerns me. This time, however, I didn't get to hear that expression. Instead, I got a few seconds of silence while he studied the mole. It reminded me how a few seconds of silence from a doctor can feel like an eternity.

Then he spoke. And he calmed all my nerves...until he didn't. He thought it might be something harmless called a seborrheic keratosis. But, he did acknowledge it was multicolored and raised and, based on my history, he thought it would be best to biopsy it. Crap! Not what I wanted to hear but the smart move.

He took a sample of the mole and told me he'd call me in a week if anything else needed to be done. Once again, I'd have to wait for the phone to ring. I made a note to invent an instantaneous biopsy.

Suffice it to say, that was a tough week. I was edgy. I downloaded a meditation app, only to delete it five minutes into my first meditation. It's fair to say I would not thrive as a monk. Who has the patience for silence?

Failing that, I actively tried to employ positive self-talk. *It probably was nothing, but even if it was something, I could handle it. I had been down that road before and came out ahead. We caught it early. Plus, God loved me and* *had my back…*which, ironically, was where the mole was.

I was truly proud of myself for fighting to stay positive. It wasn't easy. I saw it as progress, and I gave myself credit for that. But hard as I tried, that pesky pessimism was hard to squelch.

I called the dermatologist's office a few days in a row to get the results, but hung up each time when the phone started ringing because it felt counterintuitive to what I learned in therapy. Again, this was progress, even if it meant I was essentially prank-calling Dr. Bernhardt and his staff.

As I waited torturously for the week to pass, one bizarre thing did happen. It was Art Basel week in Miami: a cool annual event where Miami becomes the center of the art universe. People from all over the world flock to South Beach to spend thousands of dollars on pieces of art they may or may not appreciate. But since other rich people are buying them, how could they not buy them too? It's so Miami.

But hey, it's a fun event so I headed down there Friday night. I went to dinner with a group of people, and the conversation turned to dating and, specifically, dating deal breakers. We went around the table sharing our ultimate turn-offs. Mine was intolerance. Other people said things like smoking, not wanting to have kids, and tardiness.

Then one girl, whom I'd never met, listed pale men as

one of her dating deal breakers. Yup, she absolutely refused to date a guy who didn't tan. Of all the things someone could do wrong in her eyes, being pasty struck her as a capital offense. She and I officially had zero chance at love.

I couldn't resist, so I brought up my story. Not in a total downer, ruin everyone's Art Basel dinner kind of way, but more like, "Hey, you know, getting a suntan isn't so healthy. You might want to slather on some sunscreen."

Her reaction caused jaws to drop around the table. She said if she ever got skin cancer, or breast cancer, or any kind of cancer she wouldn't fight it. No chemo, no radiation, no nothing. She'd just cash in her chips, let it happen, and wait around to die. Mind you, this is a 30-year-old woman with her whole life in front of her. And after I tried to reason with her, it got more uncomfortable.

She added that sunscreen was more dangerous for you than the sun or tanning beds because of all its chemicals. Before I had time to regurgitate my pizza onto the table, she added that one of the reasons Americans have so much cancer is specifically because of the chemicals in sunscreen and that she'd rather take her chances with the sun.

In that moment she may have fallen in love with me because my face turned bright red. I always get mad when people say that about sunscreen. If you're so concerned, get an organic sunscreen. But do something. It's a largely preventable cancer. Try and prevent it!

I've never seen or heard from that girl again. But if I ever need to find her, I know where to look: at the beach or in a tanning bed. Yet another South Beach cautionary tale.

CHAPTER 33

Sweating The Results, But Not The Small Stuff

The seven days wore on, and no matter how hard I tried I struggled to find peace. I wasn't at previous meltdown levels, but I certainly felt tightly wound. If DEFCON 1 meant nuclear war, let's say I hovered around DEFCON 3. Not quite in crisis mode but certainly not laughing it up at an open mic night. In fact, a few times I snapped at my coworkers. Some of the blame fell on me and some of it fell on them. All right, fine, most of it fell on me.

I saw a colleague in the hall and asked her how she was doing. A simple question and one I expected would result in her saying "fine" and both of us going about our business. After all, when a colleague asks you how you're doing, aren't you just supposed to say "fine" and keep walking? Isn't that one of those societal norms? Nobody truly cares how their coworkers are doing. Don't we all know this?!?

This coworker took my pleasantry as an invitation to initiate a full-on bitch session. She hated her job, her boyfriend, the commute to see said boyfriend, felt annoyed because she didn't have any weekend plans, and believed there was "never anything fun to do in South Florida."

I took the bait. I had to contradict the last point as well as offer her relationship advice. Getting relationship advice from me is analogous to getting fashion advice from, well, me. To think, I wanted to be a matchmaker back in the day. That would have been as successful as monkhood.

That painful conversation took minutes, if not years, off my life. Please understand, I'm not typically grumpy or short with people. I happen to love people. It's part of my job. But, that week I wanted no part of any conversations. I just wanted my phone to ring with the all clear from the dermatologist's office.

It was a comment made by one of my interns later that week put everything into perspective. By Thursday my nerves were fried. This was the day I was supposed to hear back from the dermatologist, and I still hadn't heard a thing. My positivity had waned. I was still doing the uplifting self-talk, still repeating my mantras, but I'd convinced myself this new melanoma would kill me after spending much of the past two years convinced the other melanoma would kill me. I was over it and totally spent. Then my intern noticed her pen had exploded in her purse. No doubt a frustrating occurrence, but probably not worthy of her reaction.

"Fuck my life," she said. "Why do bad things always happen to me?"

She considered her pen exploding inside her Prada bag a tragedy. I don't know where she summoned the strength to go on with her day. She's a true inspiration to humanity.

I processed what she said, took a deep breath, and laughed—completely at her expense. And I felt great. As I laughed a revelation came over me. Three years ago, I might have said something similar. But now, exploding pens, flat tires, people who talk during concerts; those things didn't bother me anymore. Without even realizing it, I had learned not to sweat the small stuff, including not sweating the sweat on my face. In that moment I felt completely liberated from the minutiae that used to trouble me. Who cared if my favorite team didn't win? The players didn't care when I had a bad day, why should I care when they had one?

One of the benefits of facing your mortality is that, consciously or not, you let go of a lot of the crap that used to consume you. Partly because you realize it's unimportant and partly because you just don't have the bandwidth to process it. It isn't important enough to matter; so, you don't pay it any mind. And that's awesome.

I've even made my peace with traffic. As I mentioned earlier, it's really bad in South Florida. But now I look at traffic as an opportunity to call some of my friends, or listen to a podcast, or just think about ways I can be productive and help others.

After my intern's breakdown, I left the office energized by my newfound freedom, went home and banged out some push-ups. As I worked out, the phone finally rang. And I got the good news I had been waiting for all week: my small business had just been approved for a $250,000 loan.

Okay, so that wasn't the news I was waiting for. I didn't have a small business, and I didn't need a loan. It was an automated call from a telemarketer. I blew off my final bit of steam by yelling at that automated telemarketer and that, too, felt good.

The lesson here is don't sweat the small stuff, unless it's a telemarketer…in which case scream at them all you want; even if they're automated.

Thursday came and went but still no phone call from the dermatologist. I had an appointment to see him in a few weeks for my regularly scheduled three-month appointment, and I decided I would just wait until then to find out. If he didn't call me that would mean the news was good.

And that letting go signaled major progress. The tide was turning!

CHAPTER 34

Other People's Cancer Stories Are Not Yours

The following week I received sad news at work. A colleague's mother passed away from cancer. We all knew it was coming, but it still hit everyone in the office hard because we were a tight-knit group and most of us had worked together for years.

Doctors diagnosed my colleague's mom with brain cancer about a year earlier, after she became disoriented and confused. They operated on her and thought they got it all and believed she would be fine. But, a few months later, the cancer came back and she got very sick. Things got so bad she told her daughter she wanted to die.

While I felt deep sadness for my colleague and her family there was an impulse to internalize her story and, to some degree, make it about myself. *If this woman could die from a recurrence, maybe I could too. She was fine, free of cancer, and then it came back and she passed away within a year. What if that happened to me?* The fact that she died of brain cancer made it even tougher for me. Of all the places my disease could spread, the brain scared me the most.

But after some soul searching I was able to gain perspective and realize that circumstance wasn't about me. It was about my friend's mother. I needed to honor that, rather than put myself through unnecessary stress and create an illogical comparison. Her cancer and my cancer had nothing in common. It was comparing apples to oranges, not apples to apples.

So I let it go. But it wasn't the first time, and it won't be the last time I've experienced that situation. If you're a cancer patient it will happen to you as well. When you're going through it, and it's all you think about, you become acutely aware of other people's cancer journeys. The first year or so after diagnosis, every single time I heard someone had cancer, or died from cancer, I needed to know the details: what type of cancer, how old were they, did they beat it before it came back? It's manageable now, but, like I said, it's still an impulse of mine.

Part of the problem is, by watching the news or listening to people talk, it can seem like cancer always comes back.

You hear so many of those stories it's easy to think it's inevitable. Never mind that it doesn't always come back and that more often than not people survive cancer; it's just that survival stories aren't the ones making headlines. Hopefully that can change.

That's the thing to remember: there are indeed plenty of survivor stories. Like my friend T.J., former President Jimmy Carter, and thousands more people. Most of the board of the Melanoma Research Foundation is comprised of stage 3 and 4 survivors. That's just melanoma—there are survivor stories everywhere.

Whatever type of cancer you may have, know that it's unique. That's why you shouldn't get too hung up on recurrence rates and survival rates, because they're just numbers based on other people. You're not a statistic; you're a living, breathing organism, and I really believe you get a say in whether you live or die. You have enough to worry about when it comes to your own cancer. Don't compare it to anyone else's. But if you do, compare it to a survivor's.

CHAPTER 35

Me And The Mole People

It was the end of December and time for my regularly scheduled dermatology checkup. I hadn't heard anything about the biopsy from a few weeks ago, so either I was fine or I'd missed a call telling me I had cancer. That seemed unlikely. I did however notice a new mole on my hairline so I added that to the list to show the doctor.

That's not an expression, by the way. I actually make a list of all the moles, pimples, and freckles I find on my body because I'm afraid I'll forget about them when I walk into Dr. Bernhardt's office. I find it helps and I recommend doing the same. Sometimes you don't think so clearly in the doctor's office.

As I sat in the waiting room, a weird feeling came over me: calmness. I wasn't nervous at all. Since this whole process started I had been nervous for every single doctor's appointment; even the dentist on the off-chance they'd find mouth cancer or tongue cancer or throat cancer or whatever. But in my dermatologist's office, two years into it, in the office where it all began, I felt totally at peace. And that was weird. Part of me wanted to be nervous because of the past few years so I actually tried summoning anxiety, but I couldn't find any. For a hypochondriac and a melanoma survivor, tranquility in the doctor's office felt wonderfully surreal.

I looked around the room at the other patients, reading their *People* magazines and thought, "They have no idea how their visits are about to go." Most of them were probably just getting routine exams, but unfortunately one of them might find out they had a cancerous mole and, if so, their whole world would soon change. It's crazy that you could be sitting in a waiting room reading about Brad and Angelia (don't act like you haven't done that), and the next thing you know you're having a mole biopsied, and then a week later you get a phone call and you have cancer. You just never know.

A few minutes later Dr. Bernhardt came out and took me into the exam room. The biopsied mole was indeed totally benign. The new thing on my hairline was harmless as well. And everything else on my body was, according to him, "flawless."

After the exam I got into my car, made the requisite

phone calls to my family to share the good news, exhaled, and smiled. The car was still parked, but metaphorically I had officially turned the corner. I felt stronger now: not perfect, but stronger. In the past, good news scared me almost as much as bad news because it meant the bad news had to be coming soon, but at that moment in my car I only knew joy; sadness for Brangelina, but joy for me.

I took the day's good news for what it was: a victory. It was another day where I got to live—healthy, happy, and not in a hospital.

CHAPTER 36

Thank You God, For This Gift

In January 2017, a few weeks after the dermatologist, I had my annual brain MRI and it was all clear. Or as my friends have joked, further proof there's nothing inside my head. My oncology appointment and blood work went great too, and I began year three, post-cancer. In April of that year I had the final round of injections from my clinical trial, and I crossed that milestone off the list as well.

In 2018, I enjoyed a year of health and happiness, although there was one scare. A CAT scan revealed a nodule on my prostate. It had nothing to do with melanoma, but could have been cancerous. It turned out to be benign, but it did lead to some anxiety and more than one invasive and uncomfortable urology exam. Just to make sure that nodule doesn't become cancerous, I get to look forward to annual invasive and uncomfortable urology exams.

As I write this today, it's July, 2019, and I remain free of melanoma and prostate cancer. And boy has my life changed for the better. In television, there's an expression called "burying the lede," (that's indeed how they spell it) and it's not a good thing. It's when you lead with secondary details and save the most important stuff for last. So I won't do that. I'll lead with the big news: I'm married and my wife and I are expecting a child!

My wife, Lindsey, is the love of my life. She's the kindest, funniest, sweetest woman I have ever known and I'm immeasurably lucky to be married to her. It took me a lot of dates to find the perfect woman, but it was totally worth it. It was an instant love affair and we were married a little over a year after we met. When you know, you know.

Lindsey means everything to me and makes me want to be the best man I can be every single day. The fact that we're married makes me realize how far I've come since the beginning of my melanoma journey. I would give up my life for her, and for our future children. And that feels awesome. Oh, and as a bonus, she's a doctor, so I get to ask her as many melanoma-related questions as I want. She truly is my dream woman.

As far as my melanoma goes, I'm still in the cancer protocol, getting scans and bloodwork. The scans are scheduled to end in a year and the bloodwork should begin to taper off as well. I know I'm still at risk of a relapse, but I'm thinking forward, not backward. Rather than picturing my death, I'm imagining the rest of my life, with my wife and children and it's truly exciting. But while I'm optimistic about the future, I remain steadfastly rooted in the present, treasuring every moment and taking nothing for granted.

My ordeal with melanoma was brutal but, you know what, I'm glad it happened. Truly I am. It really did change me for the better. It's made me tougher, humbler, and more willing and eager to love. Of course, if it returns, disregard everything I just said.

I'm acutely aware that not everybody survives this disease. Many of you reading this have lost loved ones to cancer and I know some of you may be facing your own mortality. I don't know what I can say that will ease your pain, so I won't even try. I'll just say please treasure every moment you have with the people you love, and don't take any of those moments for granted.

Cancer has taught me so much. I used to be a workaholic, and I still work quite a bit, but when I got the phone call that I had melanoma the last thing on my mind was how much money I had made. You don't wish for more money;

you wish for more time.

Cancer has also taught me what I need to work on with myself. Clearly, I don't always respond well to stress, and I'm still prone to neurosis and hypochondriasis. I'm making strides. For me, laughter is the key to the whole thing. Trying to find the humor in every situation is the best coping mechanism for me. Hopefully it's a source of strength for you as well.

I'm also learning to take life slower and to enjoy the little things. I make a conscious effort to take my time eating so I can appreciate every single bite. Except with pizza; I still scarf that down. Eating slower may sound silly but, believe me, it really enhances your enjoyment of the meal.

I'm finding joy in experiences I never cared about very much. I've seen my share of sunsets and even a few sunrises and saw an amazing double rainbow this morning. At least I think it was a double rainbow: I am color-blind, after all.

Professionally, I've started a Media and Public Speaking Coaching business. I'm helping people overcome their fears of public speaking and giving them the confidence and skills they need to thrive on camera, on stage and in one-on-one settings. I've also interviewed a ton of incredible people over the past few years on television, including John Travolta, Halle Berry, former Vice President Al Gore, and many more. Not to mention all the doctors I've interviewed about various cancers and what our viewers can do to prevent them.

I've even treated myself to a dream vacation three years in a row. Every January, two of my best friends and I play in a one-week Major League Baseball Fantasy Camp in Phoenix, Arizona. It's the vacation of a lifetime—playing baseball with friends while former major leaguers coach us—but one I would have probably never taken in the past. It's pretty expensive so I would have passed on it, or put it off for "another year." Now I know you're not guaranteed another year. You're not guaranteed anything beyond this moment. So, the plan is to keep going to baseball camp and to go on more dream vacations with my wife and family. Life is wonderful and I feel like my eyes are truly open and I can live fully.

That's only part of the journey for me. In order to live my life to the fullest, I need to completely turn my "cancer problem" into my "cancer opportunity." How can I use what happened to me as a way to save lives? Many people with stage 3 melanoma die, but not me. I'm here and I'm not wasting that blessing.

As I mentioned, I truly believe God gave me cancer

because of my ability to communicate, whether that is on television, as a public speaker, as an author, or just some guy at the beach asking strangers if they're wearing sunscreen. The reason I am alive is to save lives. If I can save just one person from getting melanoma, or convince one person to get a suspicious mole checked, I think I've earned the gift of life. But I plan on impacting way more than just one person. I want to help get legislation passed that bans tanning beds. I want to make sunscreen mandatory for every child playing organized sports. That's just the beginning.

I want to be more than an advocate in the fight against melanoma; I want to be the face of the disease. My goal is to share my story nationally and do my part to raise enough money so we can cure melanoma, once and for all. And with this book, I want cancer patients to know there is a community of people here to help, and you should lean on them. I did, and it made a world of difference.

And remember, it's okay to be scared. You'd be nuts if you weren't, so don't beat yourself over it. Just try to laugh as often as you can (even if it's at yourself) and keep your head held high. You're a warrior just for being in the fight. You've got this. Just keep taking it one day at a time.

I'm very much a work in progress, but that's okay—it's

who I am. If that's who you are, that's okay too. Now go outside, run around, and have fun…but first, put on your hat and sunglasses and apply SPF 30 with UVA and UVB protectant! Enjoy!

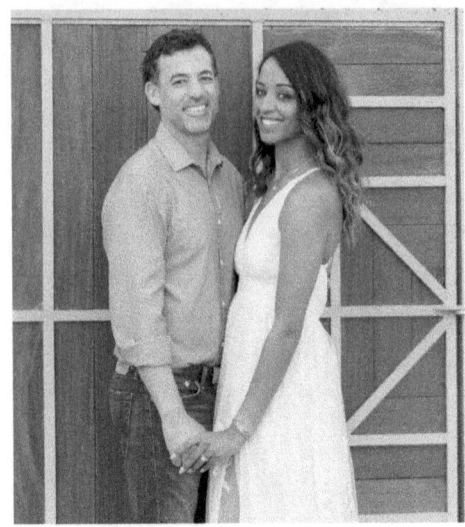

My beautiful wife, Lindsey.

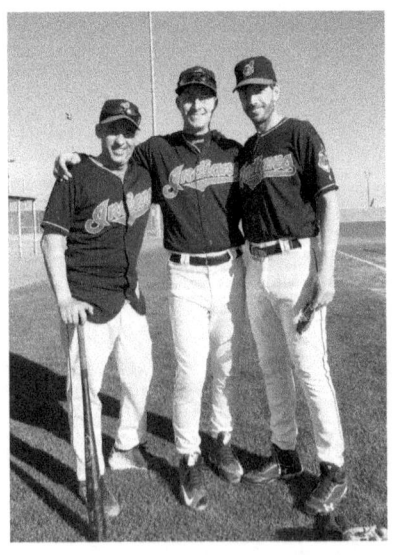

Cleveland Indians Fantasy Camp with my
buddies, Jeff and Josh.

Thank you so much for reading my book. I hope it's inspired you to soak up as much joy (but not sun) as you can from every day of your life.

Life is a wonderful blessing and it should be celebrated. If you'd like to learn more about me, or if you wish to contact me, just visit **www.daveaizer.com.**

Thank you!